Colors of Health

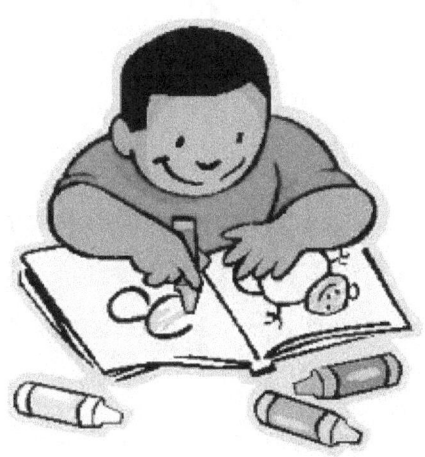

*Art for Well Body and Mind *

By Melvia F. Miller

Colors of Health

Art for Well Body and Mind

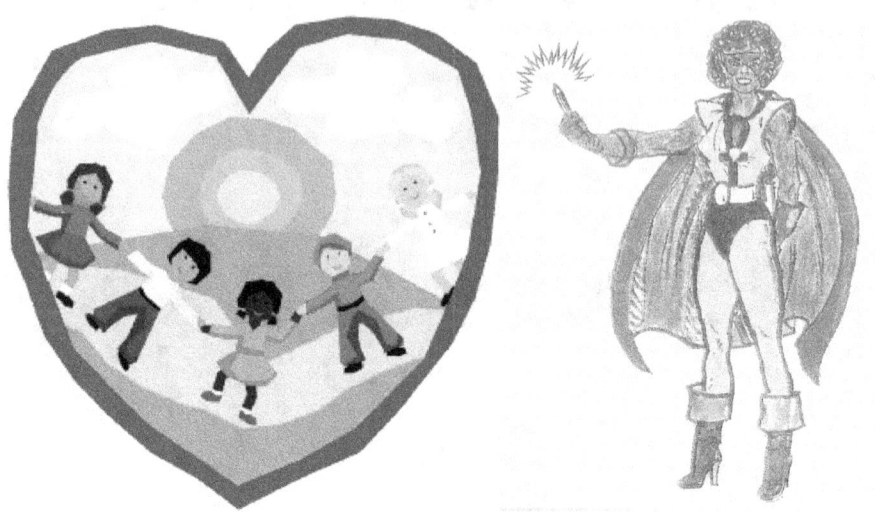

Published by **Edutainment Enterprises**

Printed in the U.S.A.

This book belongs to: _____

Phone = ___(_____)_____

HEALTH COLORING BOOK
FOR YOUTH

PLUS—

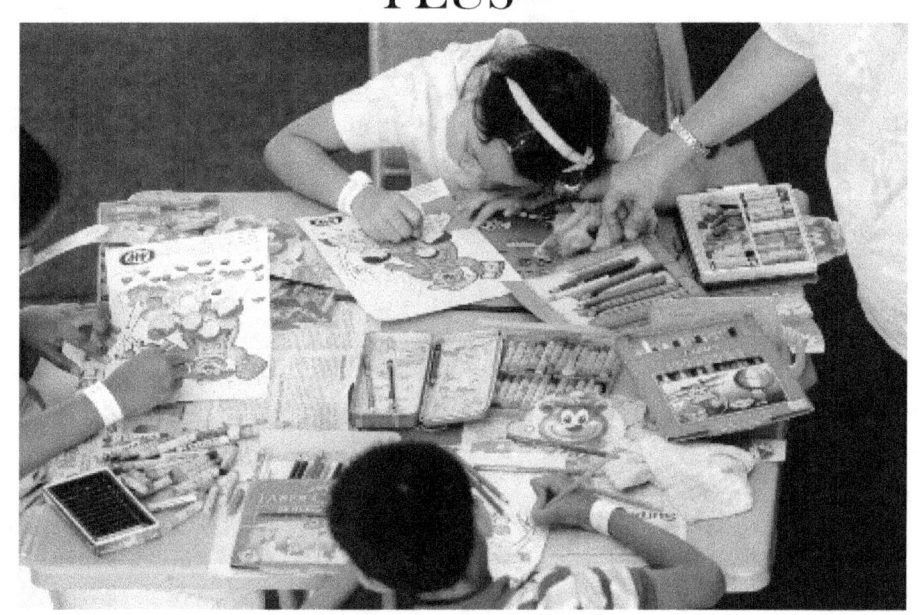

EDUTAINMENT
ACTIVITIES

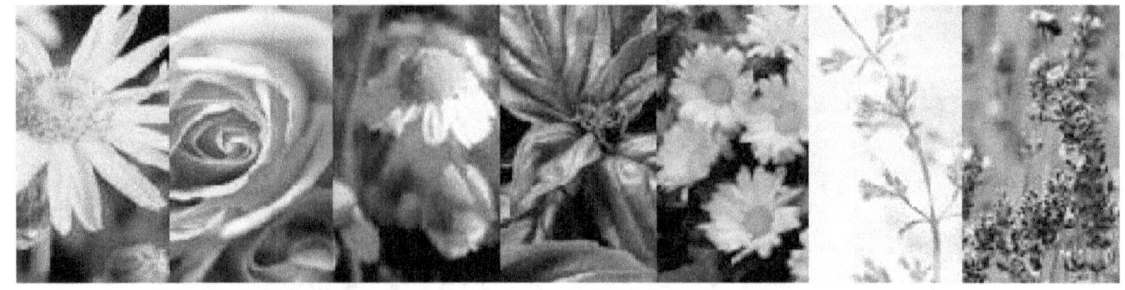

All praise and thanks are due to "the Great Spirit" for blessing me with the talent, skills, and education to compose this book.

DEDICATION:

This book is dedicated to my 2 wonderful sons, Malik and Mikal, who have been the light and delight of my life. My sons are very special people and will receive most of the benefits, proceeds and honors derived from the sales of my books. I could not have accomplished the completion of this book without my 2 sons.

THANKS:

A SPECIAL THANKS TO MY MOTHER AND FATHER for raising me. I could not have accomplished this writing project without the help, support and love of all of my many friends. I deeply appreciate all of the people who have assisted me in various ways throughout my life.

~Melvia F. Miller *(aka: "the Soulful Dr. Seuss)*

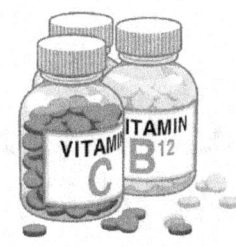

Contents

IT IS TIME FOR US ALL TO GET HEALTHIER AND HAPPIER

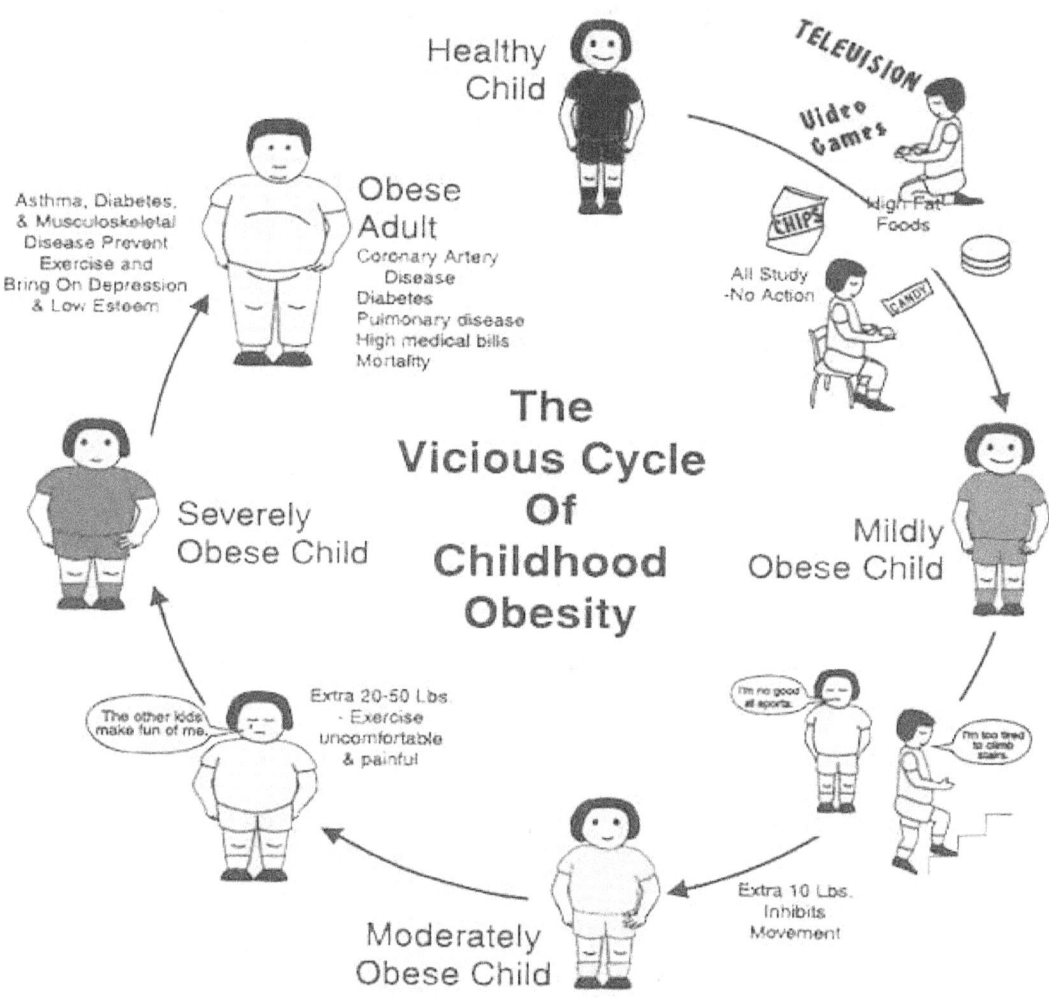

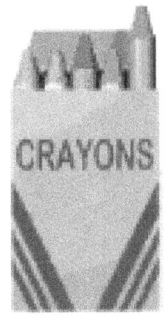

EDUTAINMENT COLORING PAGES
...and ACTIVITIES

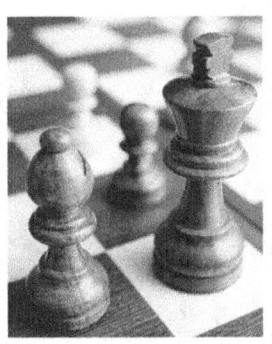 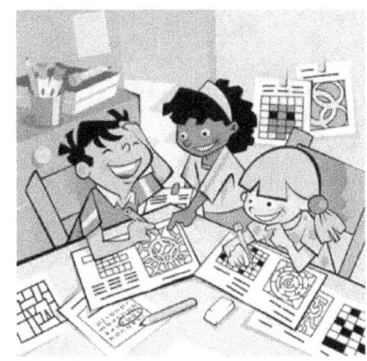

"A wise teacher makes learning enjoyable...."

Created by Author Melvia Miller, who specializes in *"Edu-tainment"*

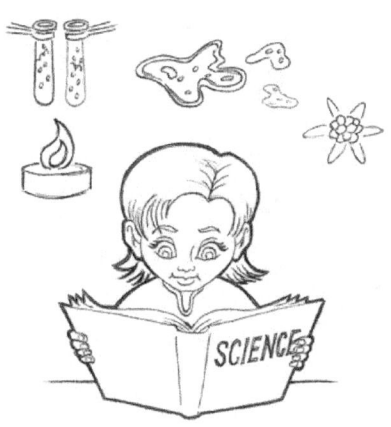 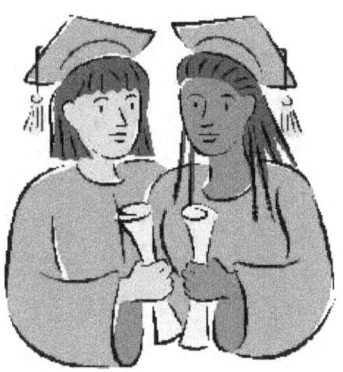

Educational Research shows that classes are most effective when

we utilize our senses, minds, hands, and are involved in activities.

The more we learn about the Natural World – the better we can understand ourselves…as we are 'the environment.'

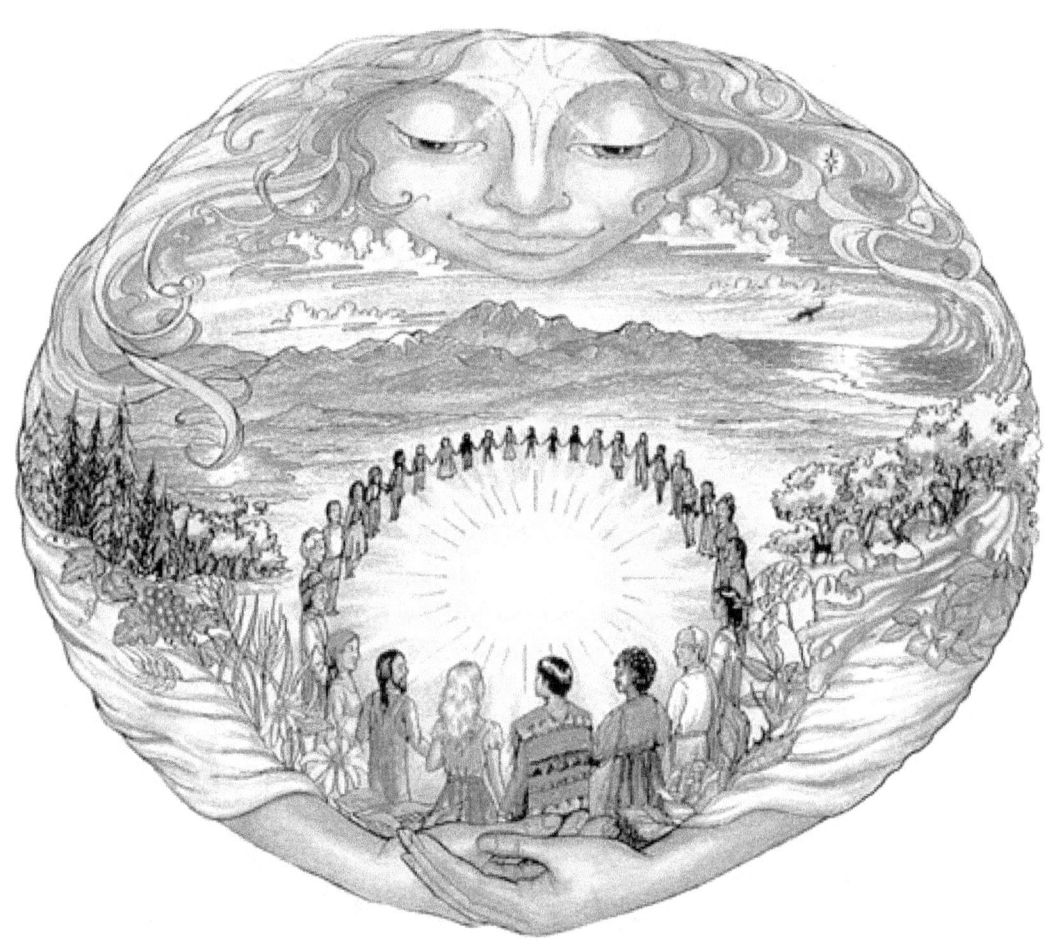

We are all connected.

ABOUT FOOD

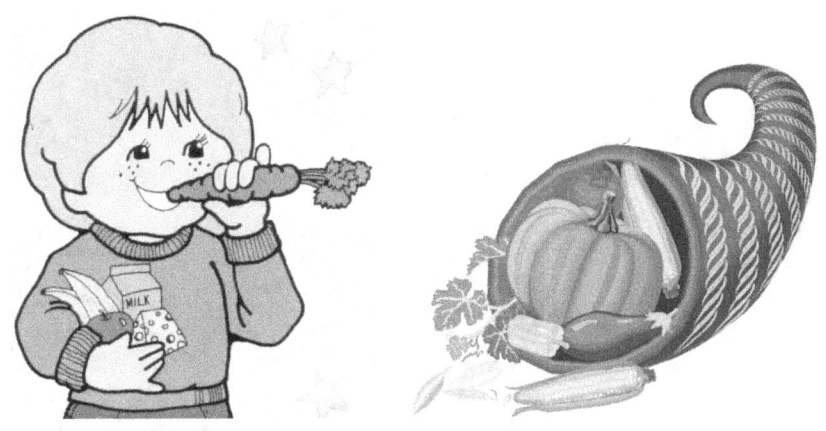

AND NUTRITION

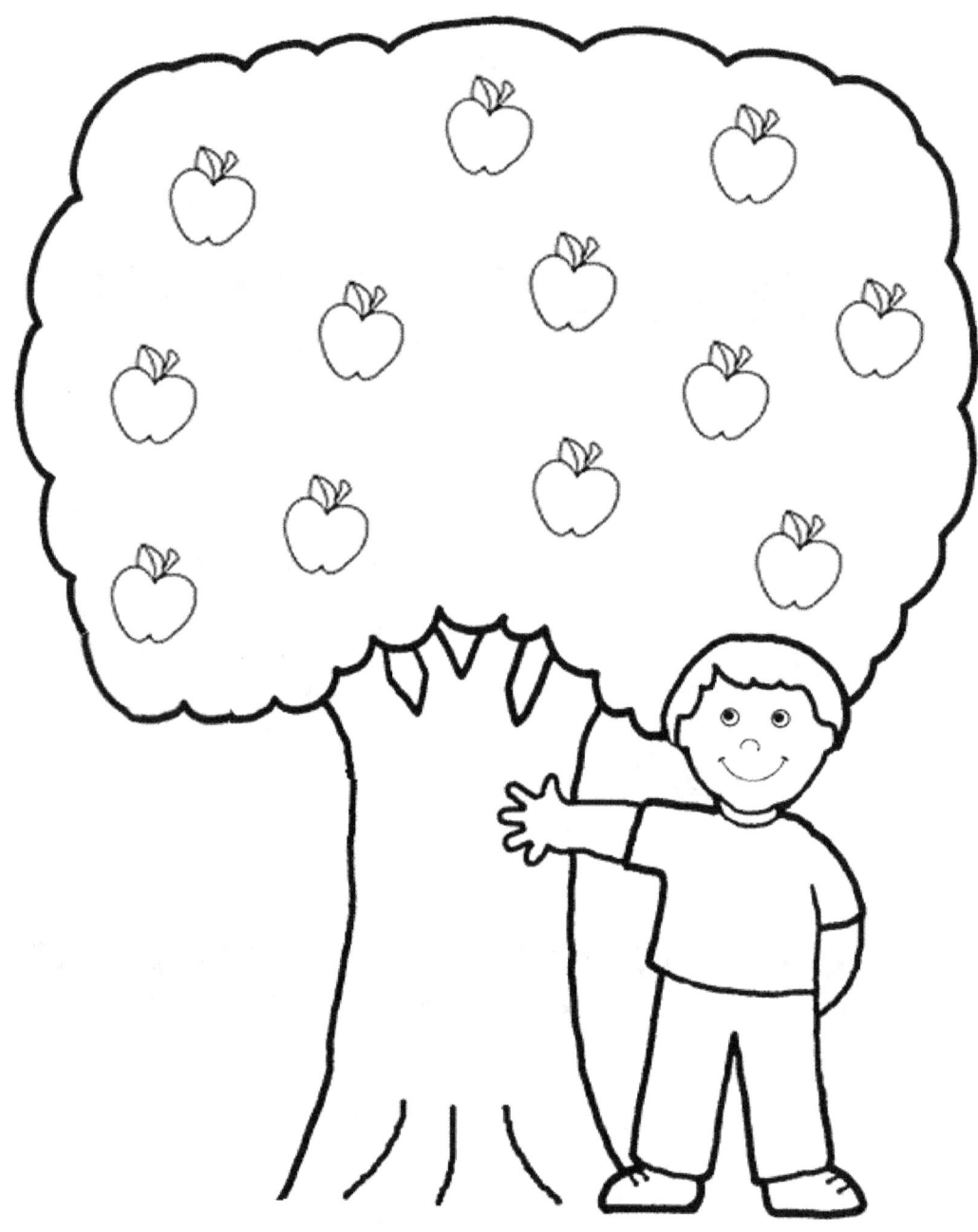

A is for _____

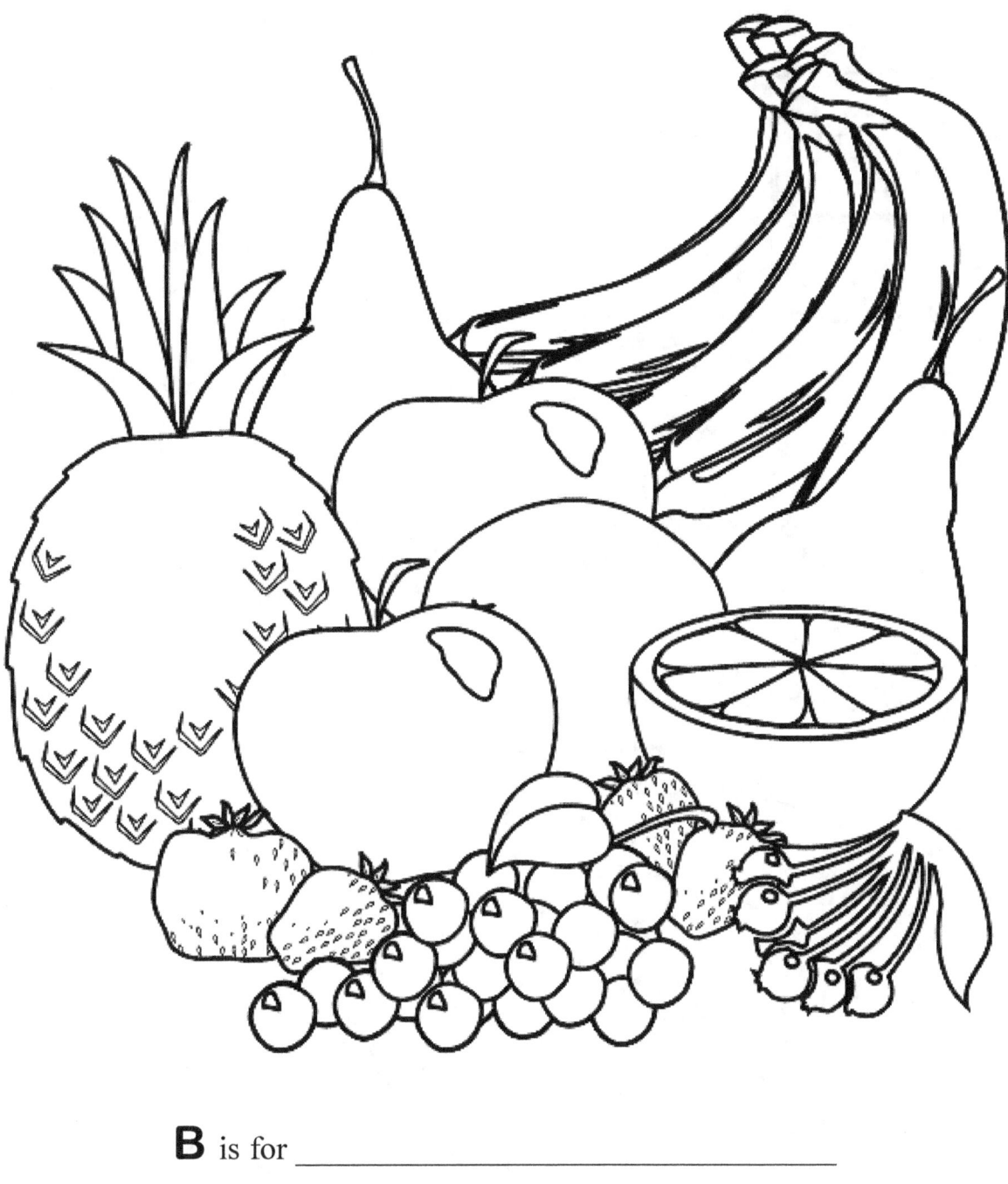

B is for _____

C is for _____

Name your favorite fruit = _____

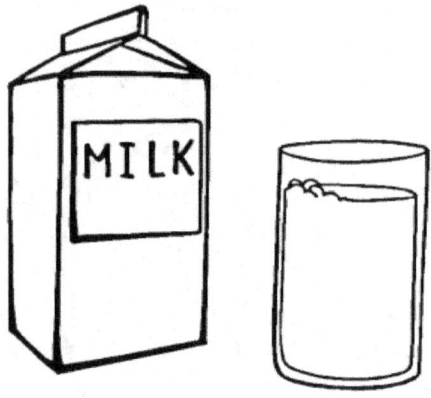

Circle the picture that shows where **milk** comes from....

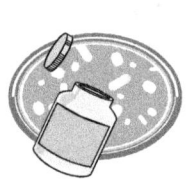 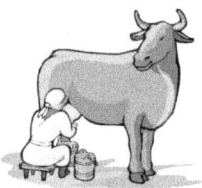 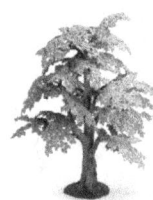 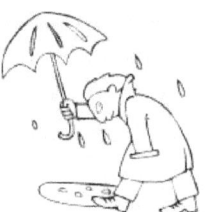

One way that milk is used is in cereal ----

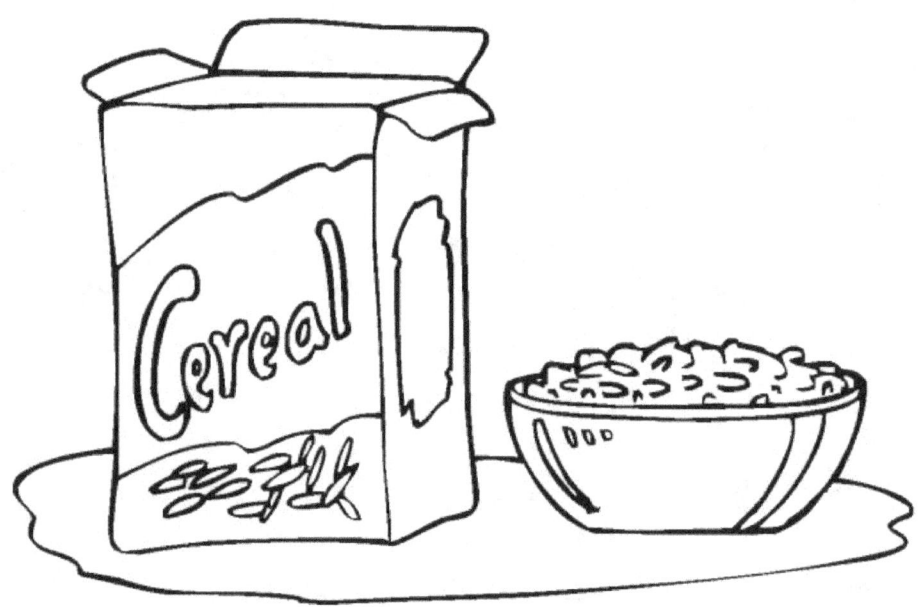

Name another way that milk is often used – _____

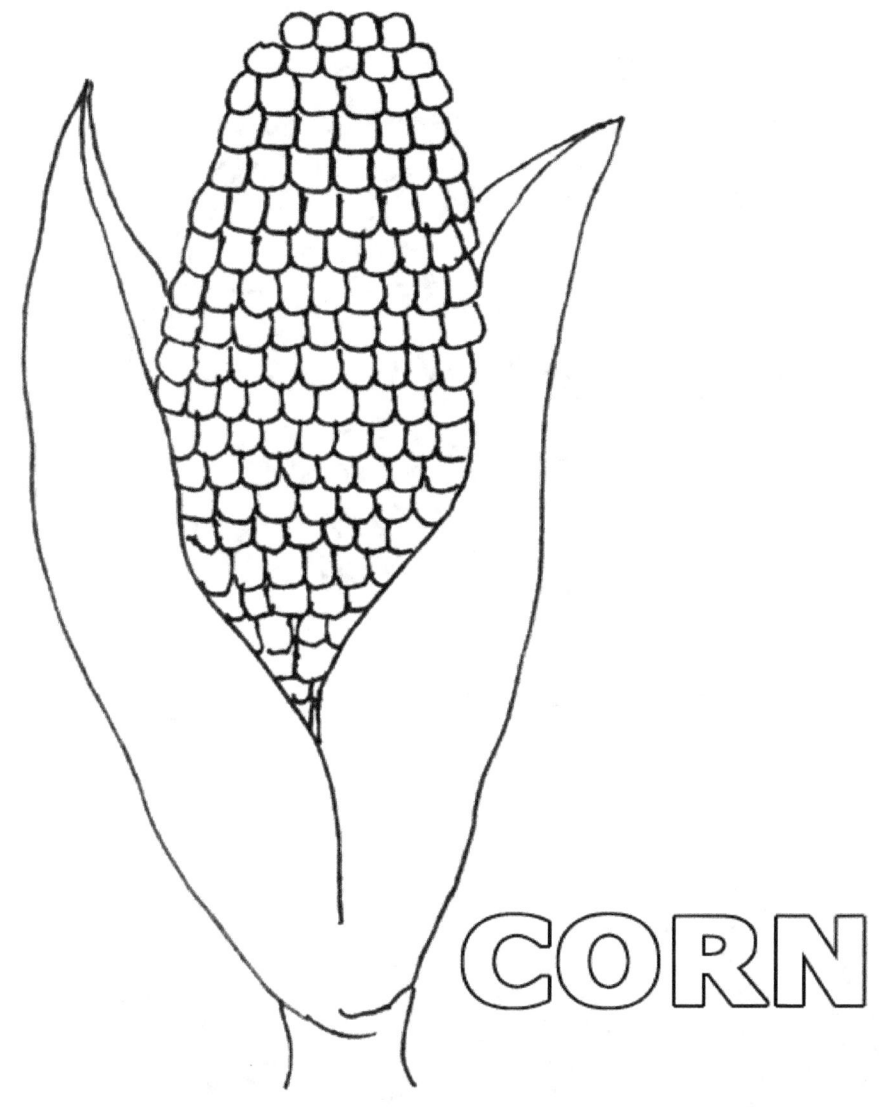

CORN

DRAW YOUR OWN SKETCH OF A FOOD THAT CONTAINS CORN...

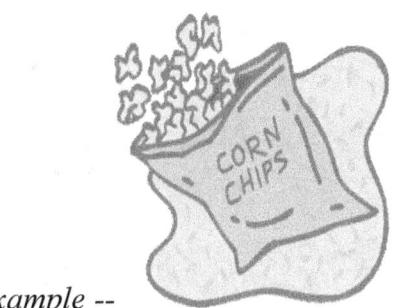

Example --

13

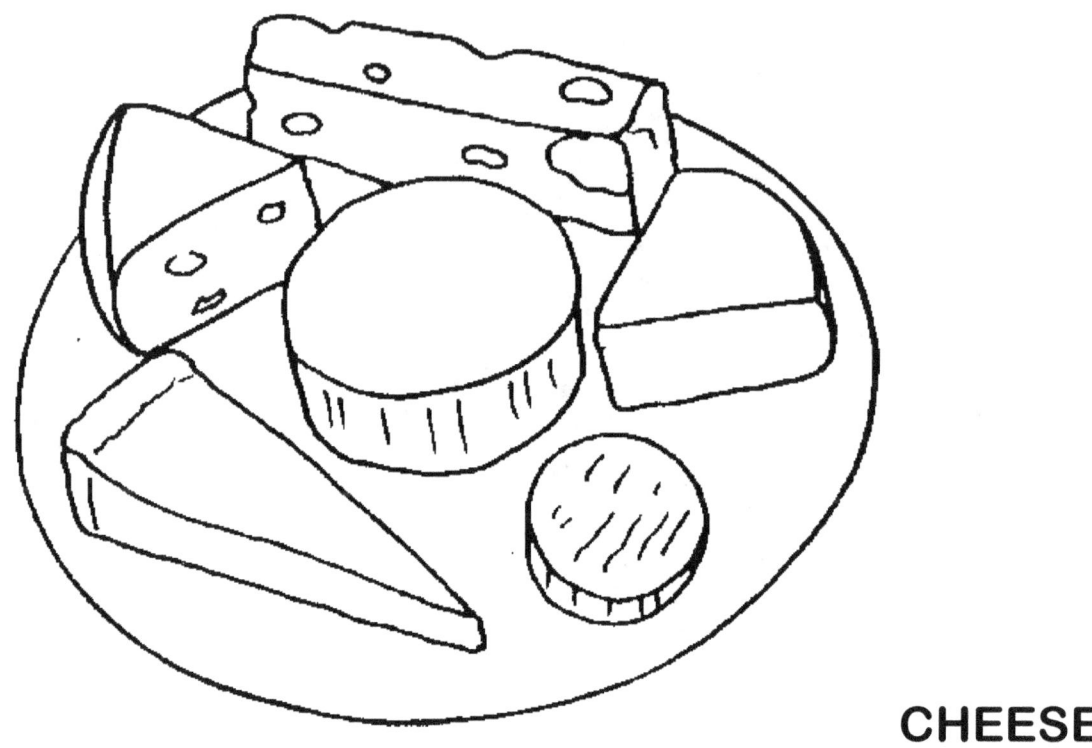

CHEESE

Put an **X** over the places where you should **<u>not</u>** put cheese —

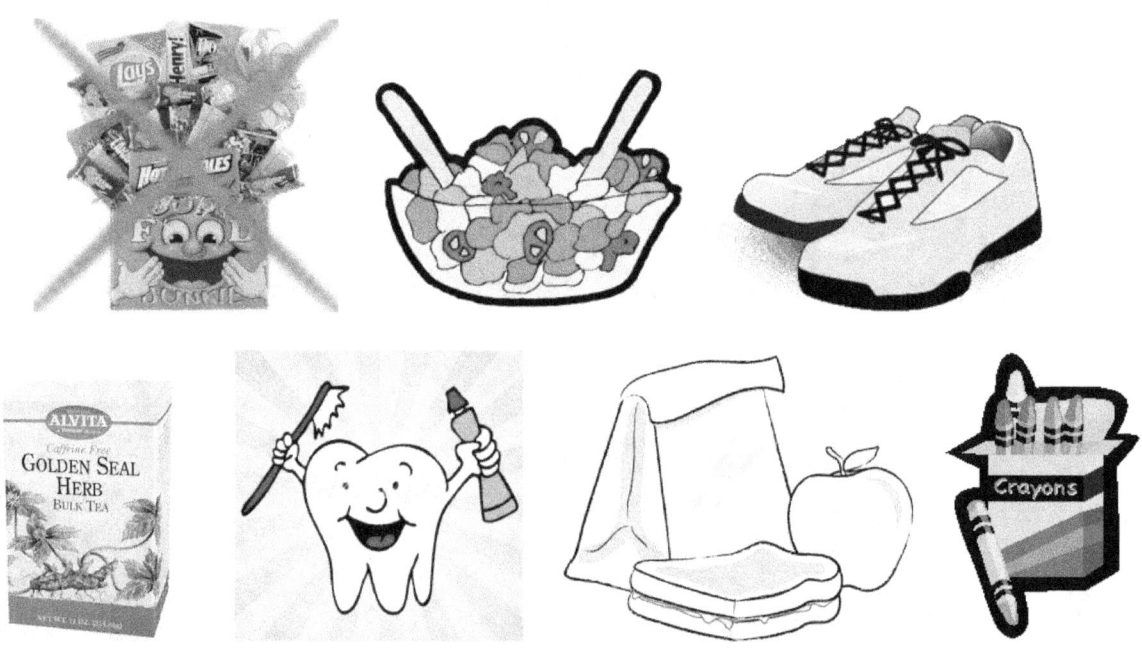

14

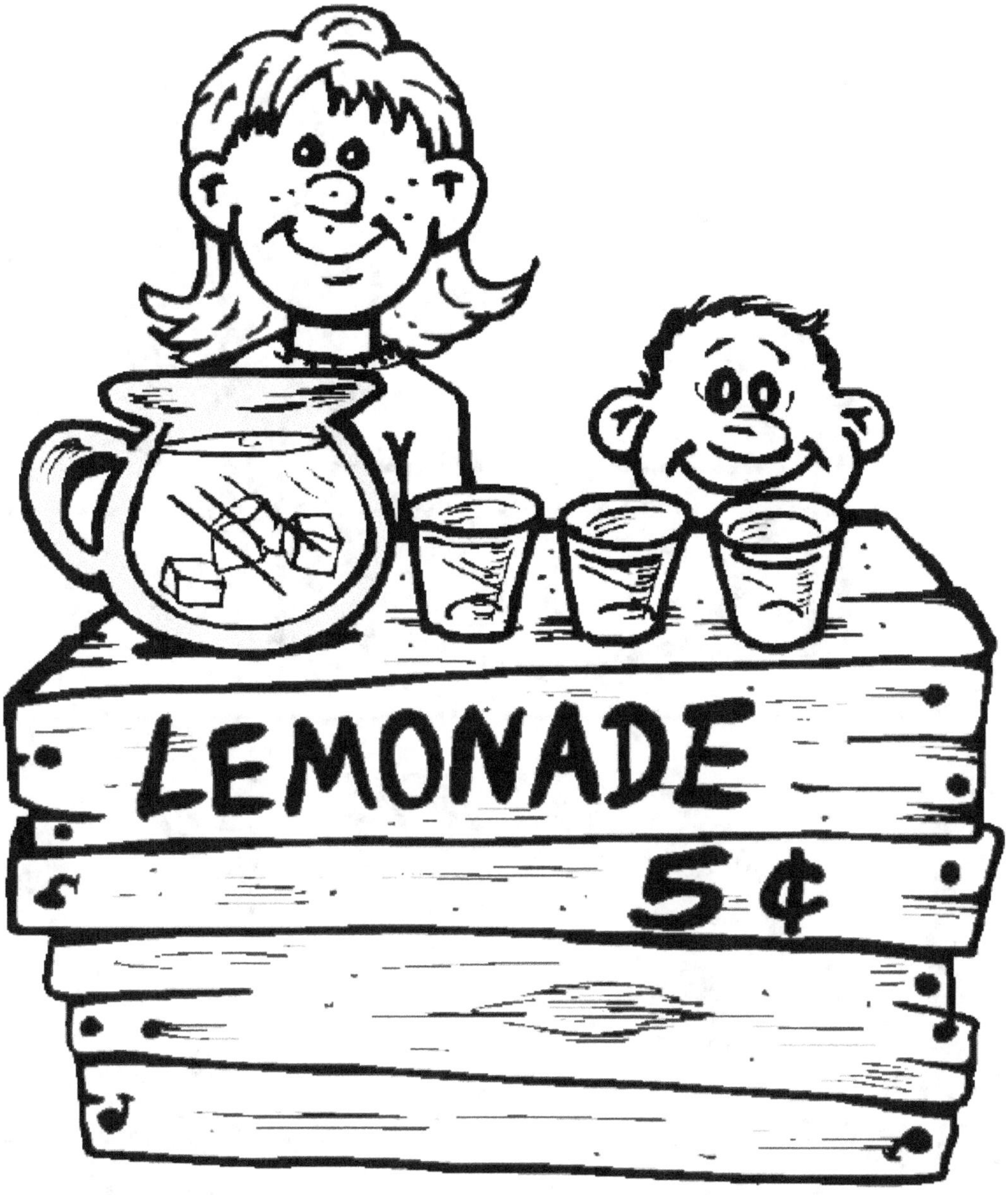

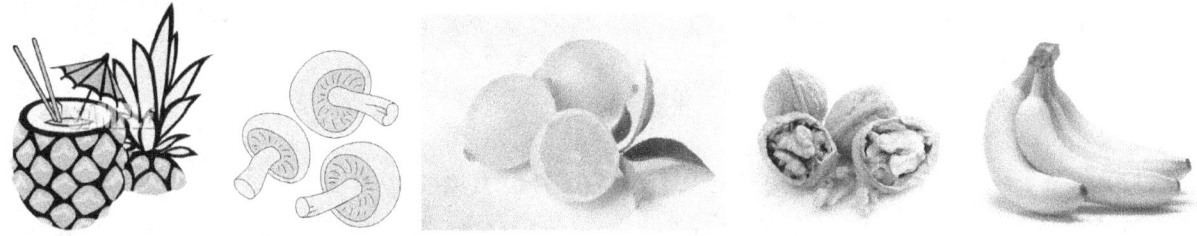

DRAW A CIRCLE AROUND THE FRUIT USED TO MAKE LEMONADE

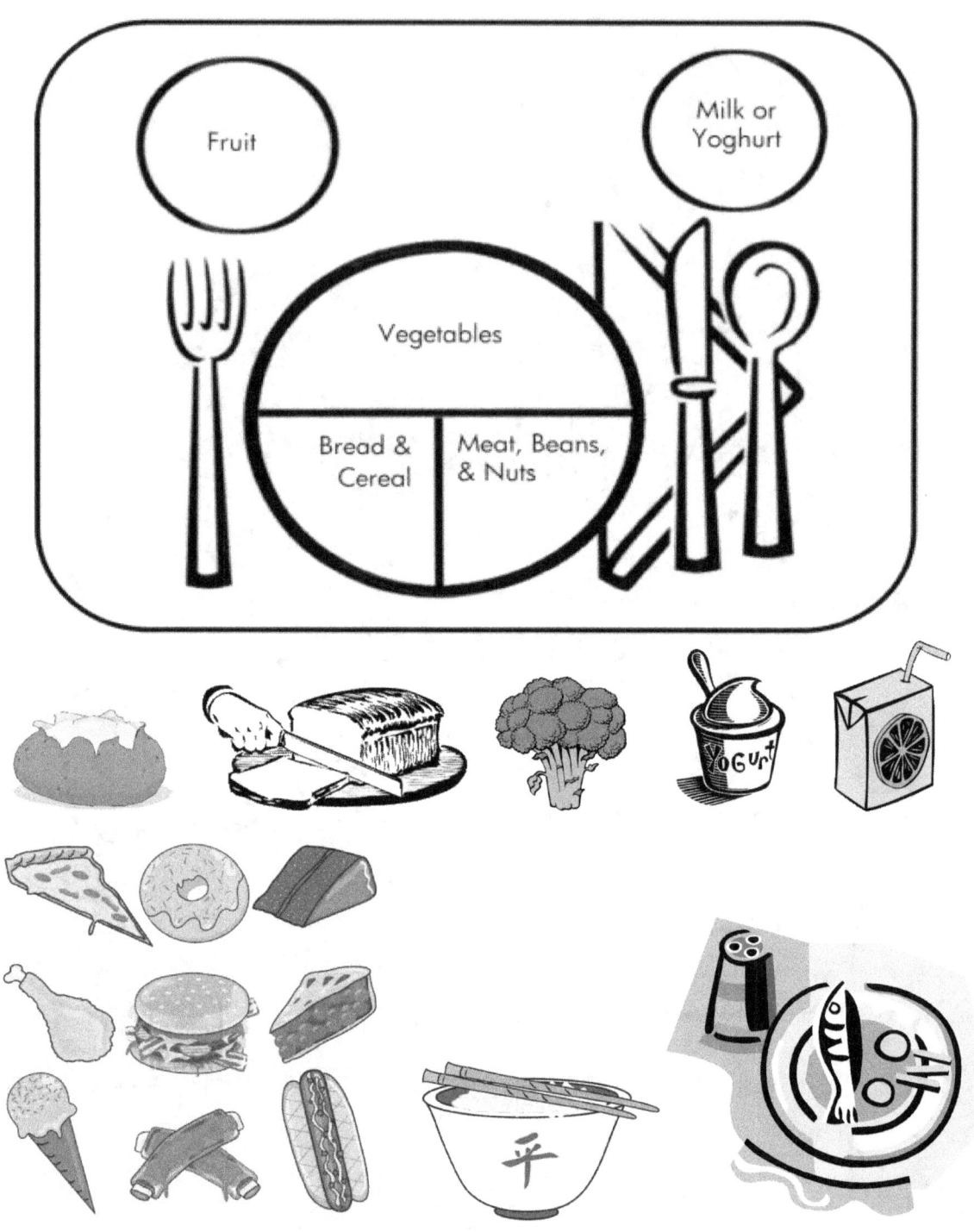

Draw a circle around the FOODS and then draw a line from the food to the plate to show what you would prepare to make a **healthy meal** for dinner.

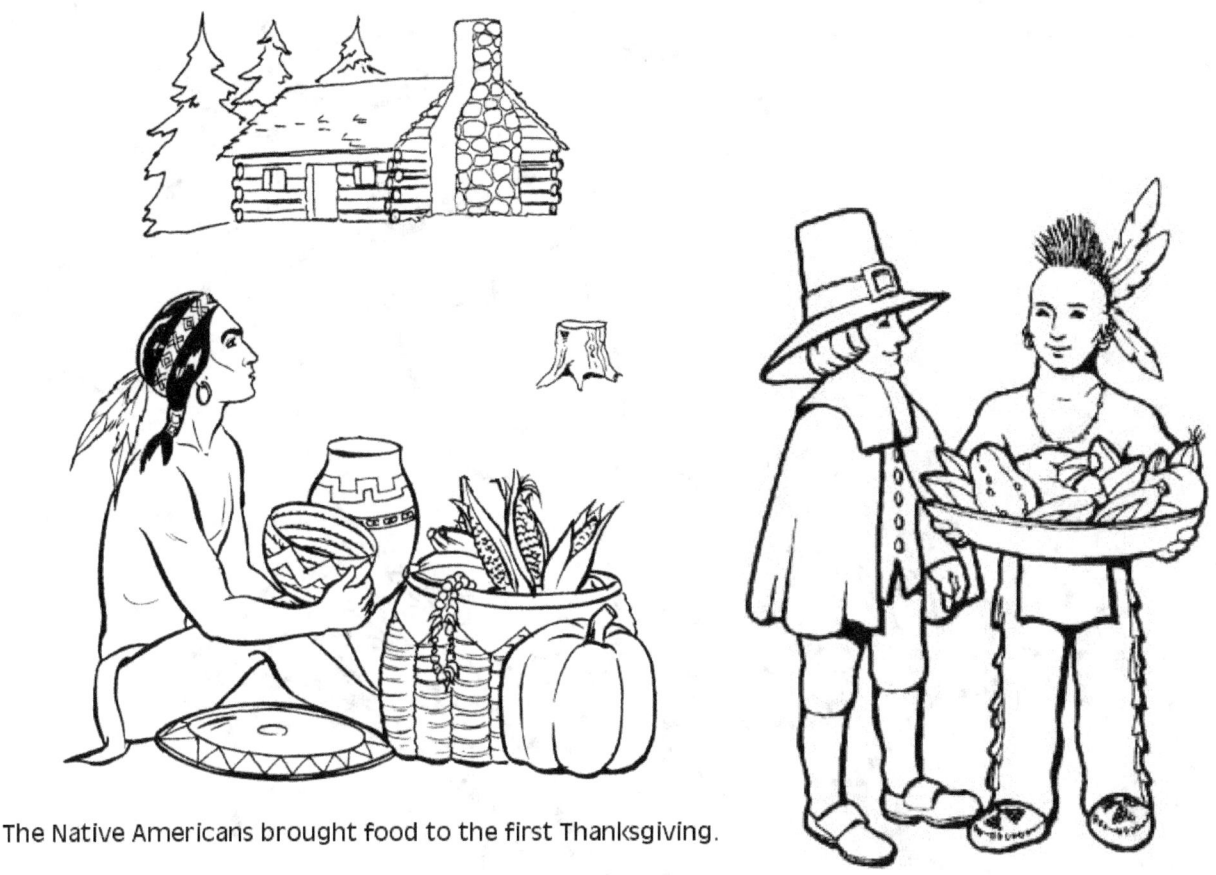

The Native Americans brought food to the first Thanksgiving.

Name 3 or 4 of some of the foods that **Native Americans** (Indians) included in their meals....

_____

_____

What did they use for medicines? _____

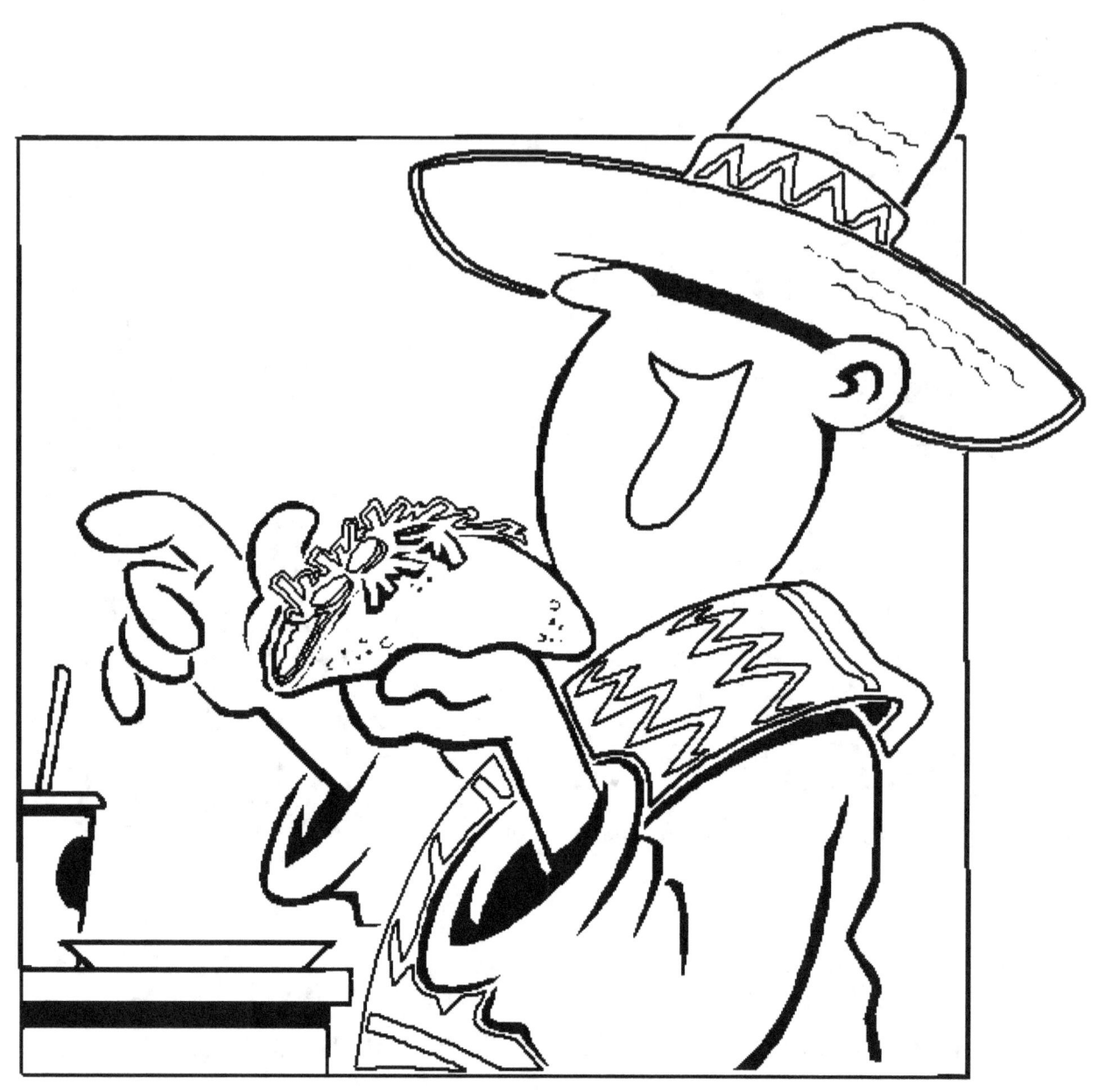

Name 2 popular Mexican foods or dishes:

_____

_____

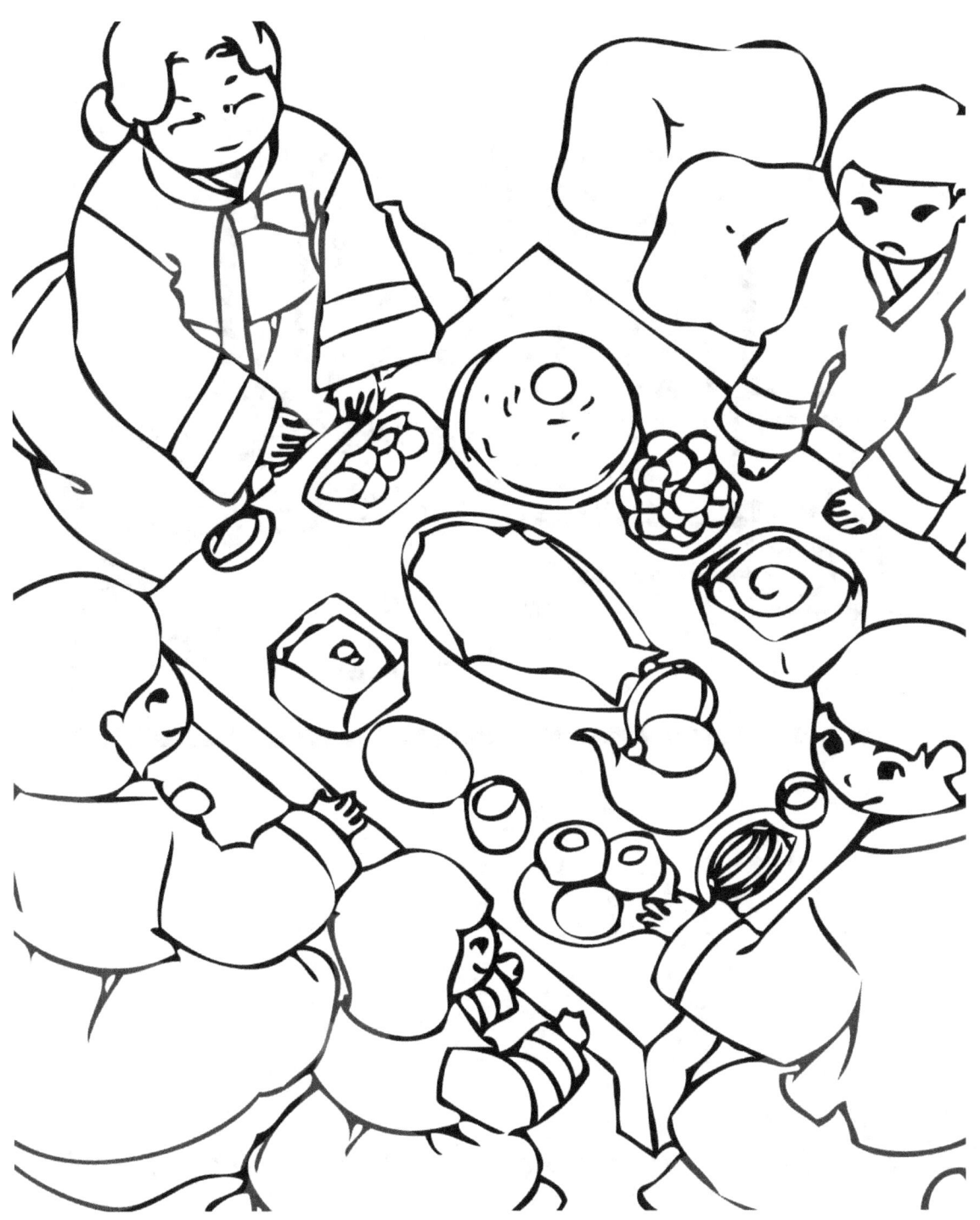

Can you name a popular food from Japan or Asia?

_____

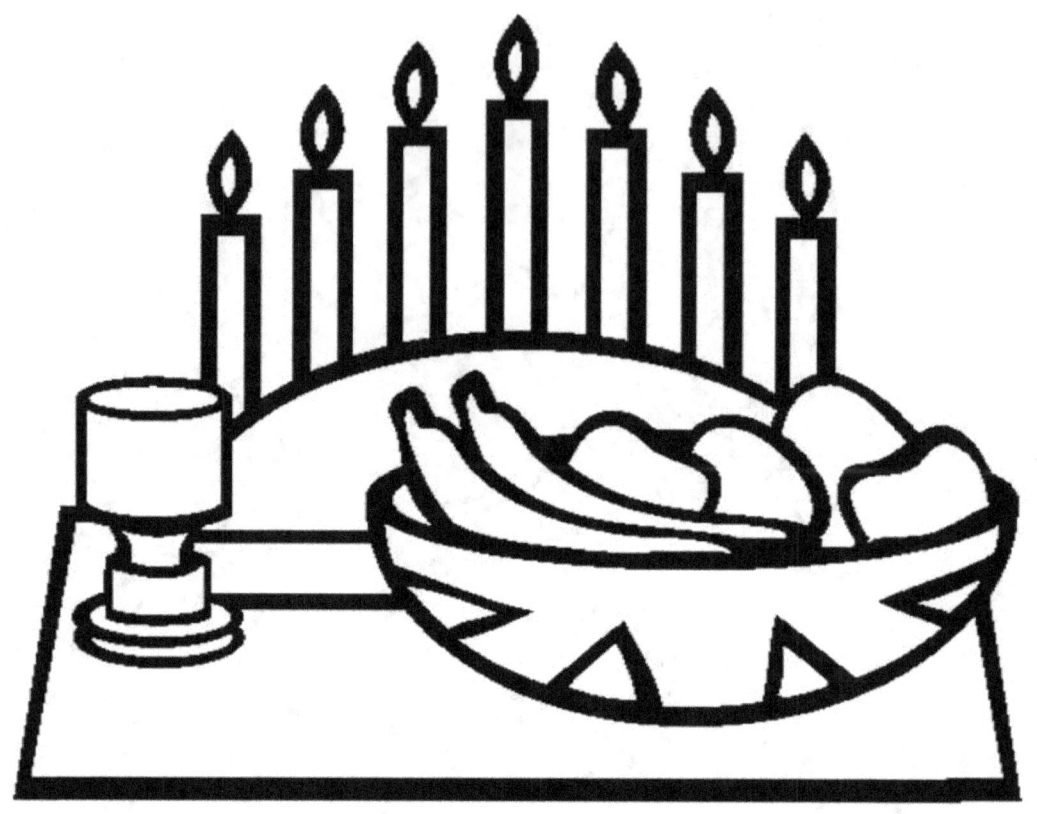

K W A N Z A A

What foods are placed on the Kwanzaa display ?

_____

Why do they use these foods? _____

ABOUT

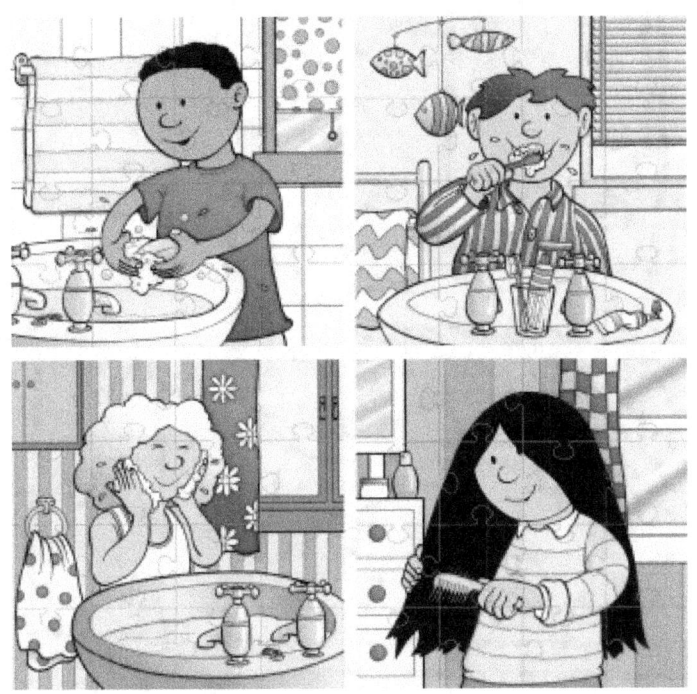

SAFETY AND

HYGIENE

Wash and dry your hands before you make or eat a snack or meal.

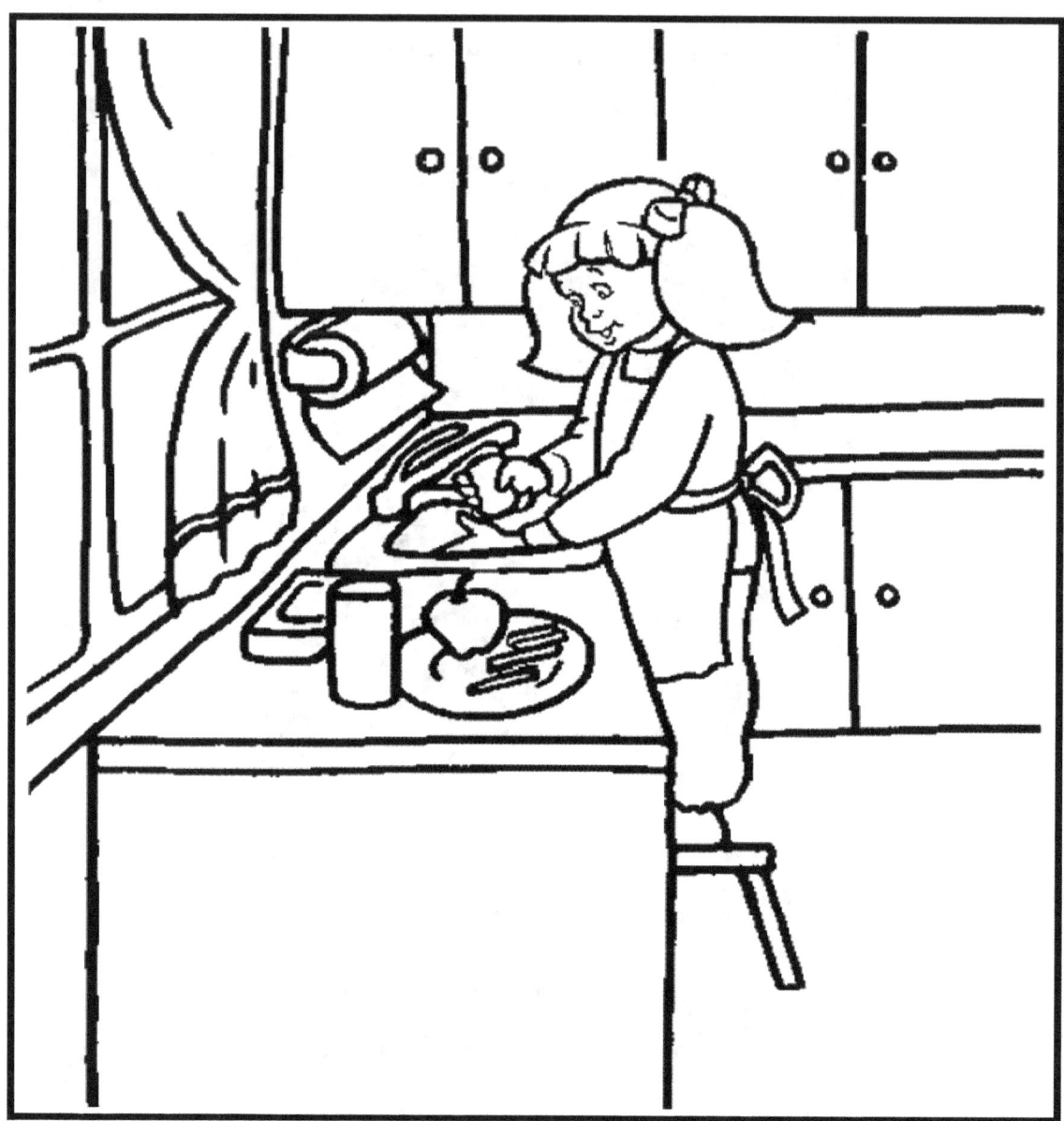

Name 2 other things that you should wash before eating _____

_____

Put foods like milk, yogurt, lunch meat and eggs back in the refrigerator right away. Don't leave them out on the counter.

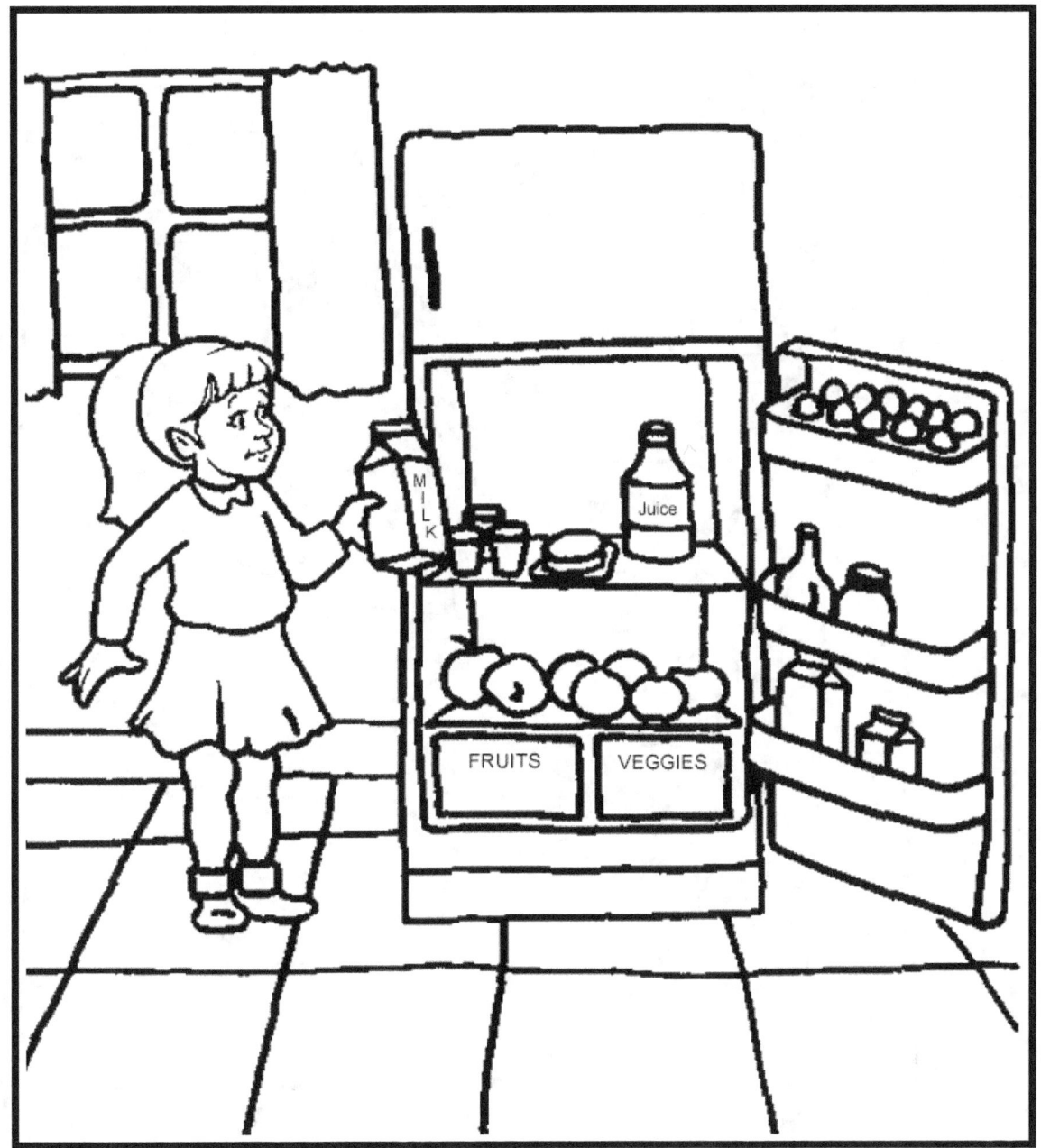

Give one reason why we should do this --- _____

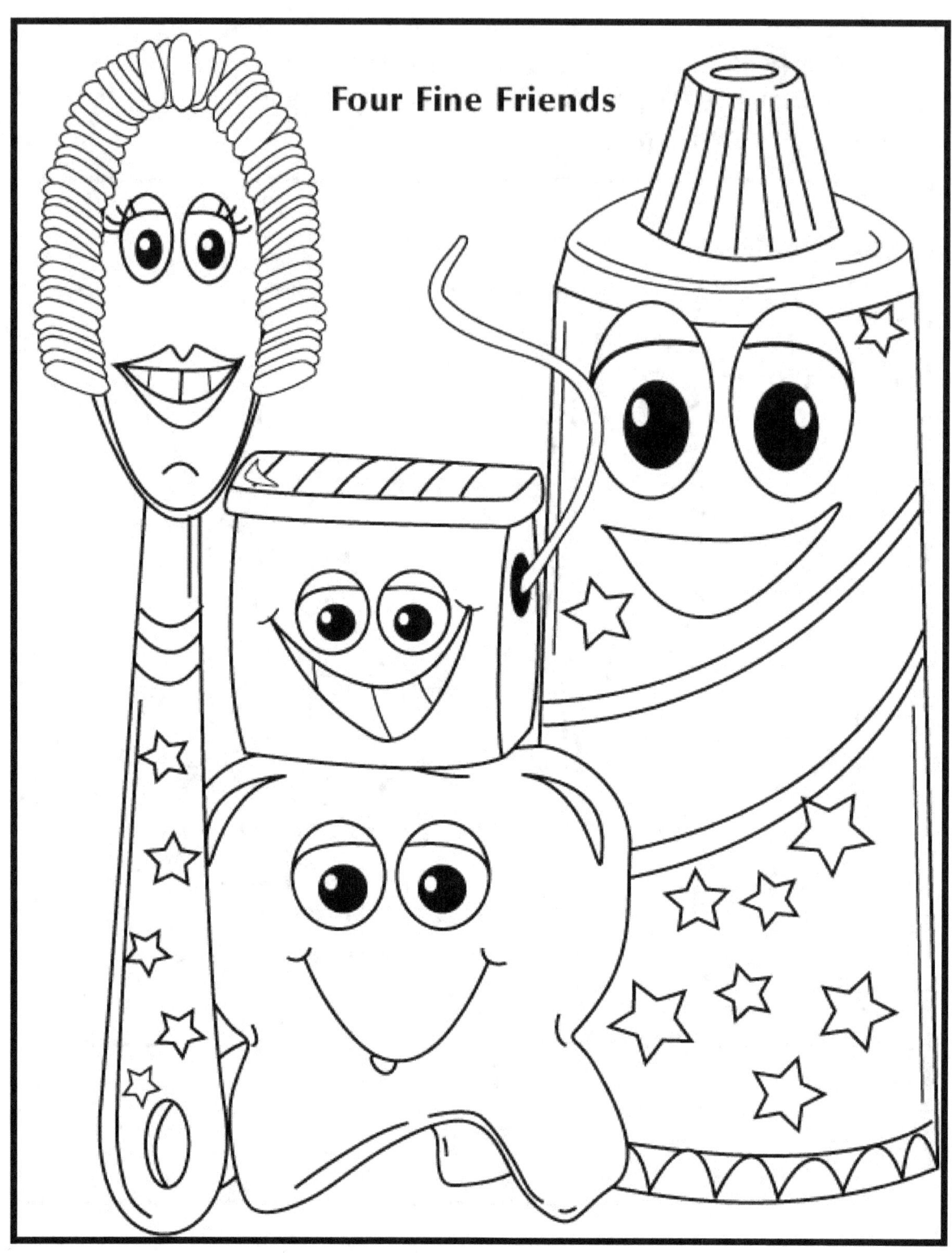

Four Fine Friends

Take turns telling other friends what you know about taking care of teeth.

24

When you pack a lunch, keep **HOT foods HOT** and **COLD foods COLD**. A thermos or an ice pack will help.

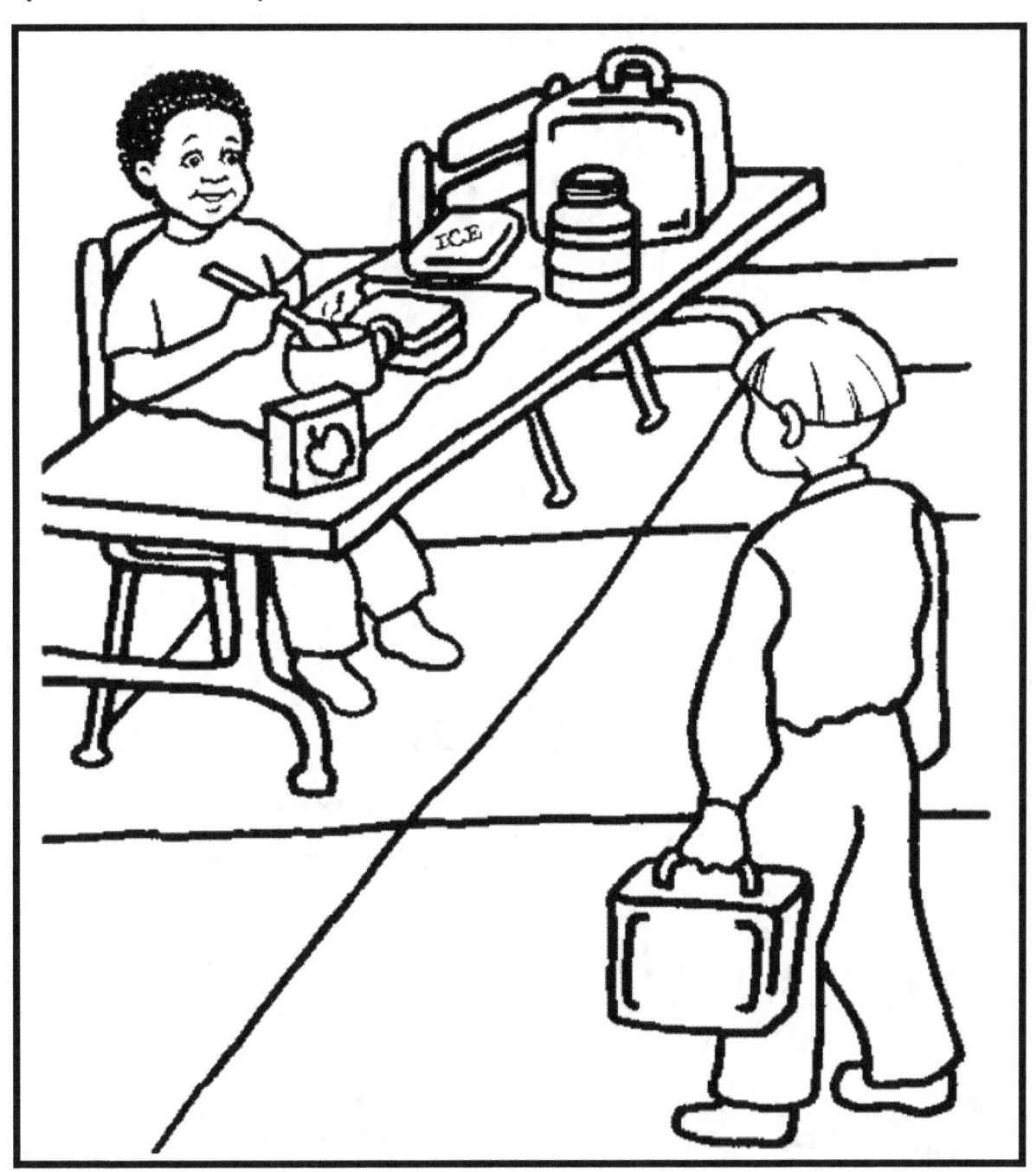

What should you do if
your clothes catch on fire?

stop

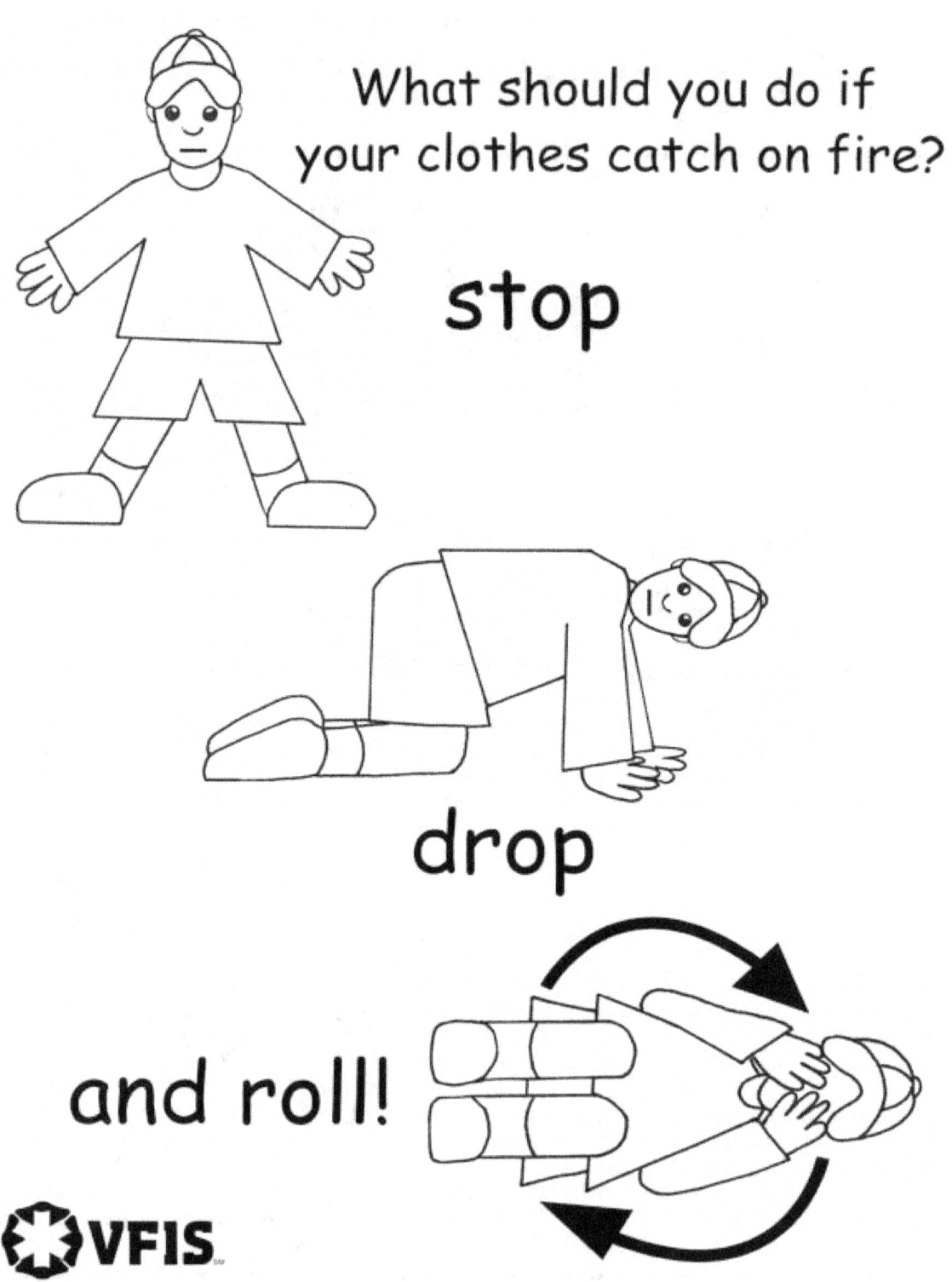

drop

and roll!

WHAT BASIC ITEMS ARE IN A **FIRST AID KIT** ?

How many can you name? How are they used?

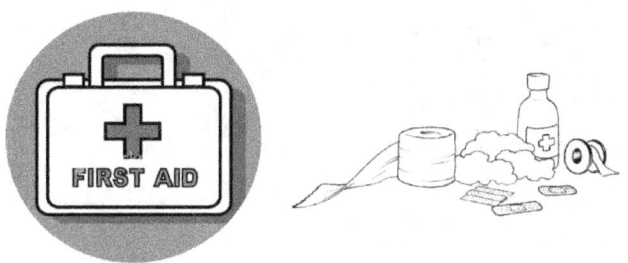

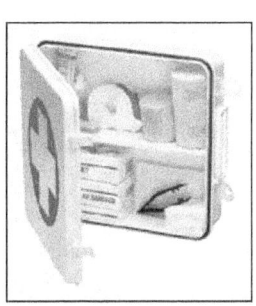
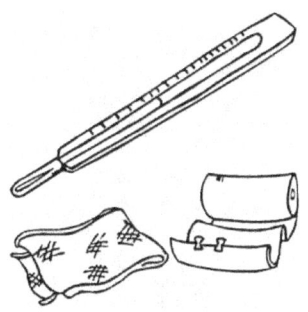

LIST 3 MORE ITEMS THAT YOU WOULD PUT IN AN EMERGENCY KIT THAT YOU WOULD HAVE IN CASE OF A DISASTER – *such as:* **power-outage, tornado, flood, etc.**

*Draw a circle around the things you <u>would</u> put in an Emergency Kit —

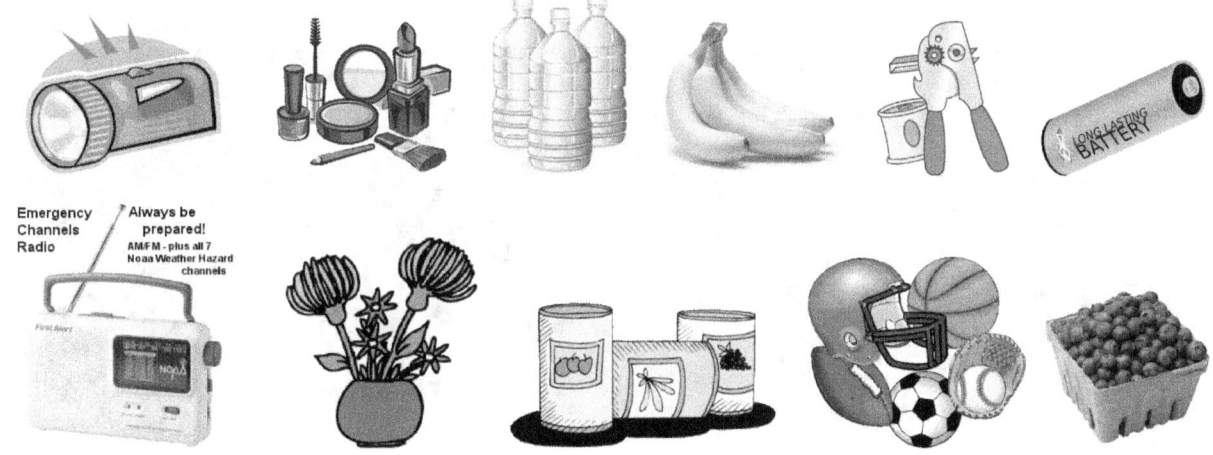

Find out what is in your food before you buy it or eat it.

 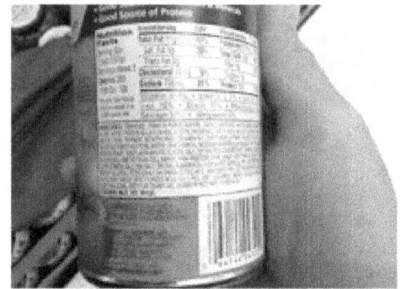

TOO MANY CHEMICALS AND ADDITIVES ARE <u>NOT</u> GOOD FOR HEALTH !

Drugs are poison...and *will kill you !*

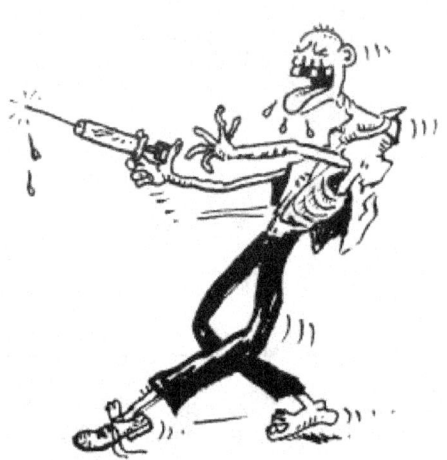

Drug addict

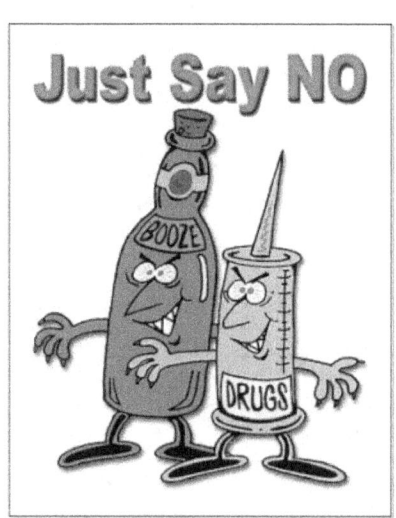

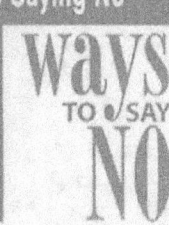

1. Saying "No Thanks"
2. Giving a Reason or Excuse
3. Repeated Refusal, or Keep Saying No
4. Walking Away
5. Changing the Subject
6. Avoiding the Situation
7. Cold Shoulder
8. Strength in Numbers

ways TO SAY NO

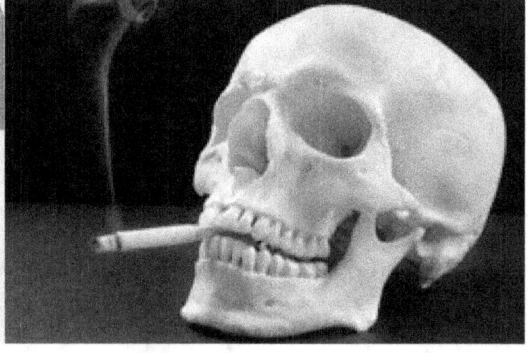

ABOUT

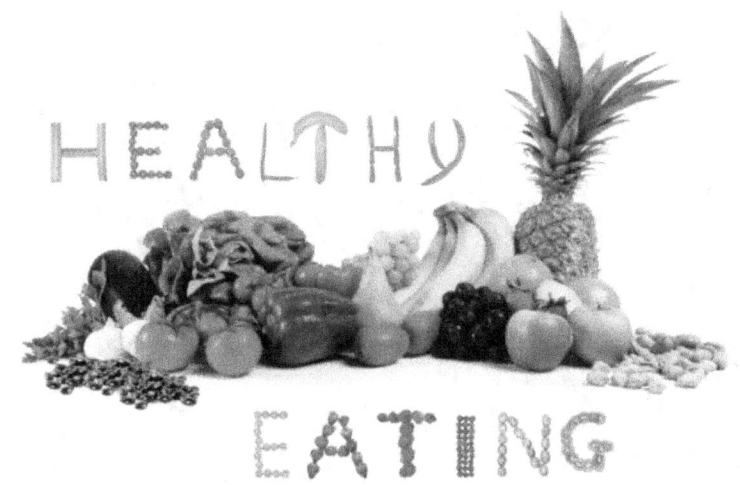

CHOICES and FITNESS

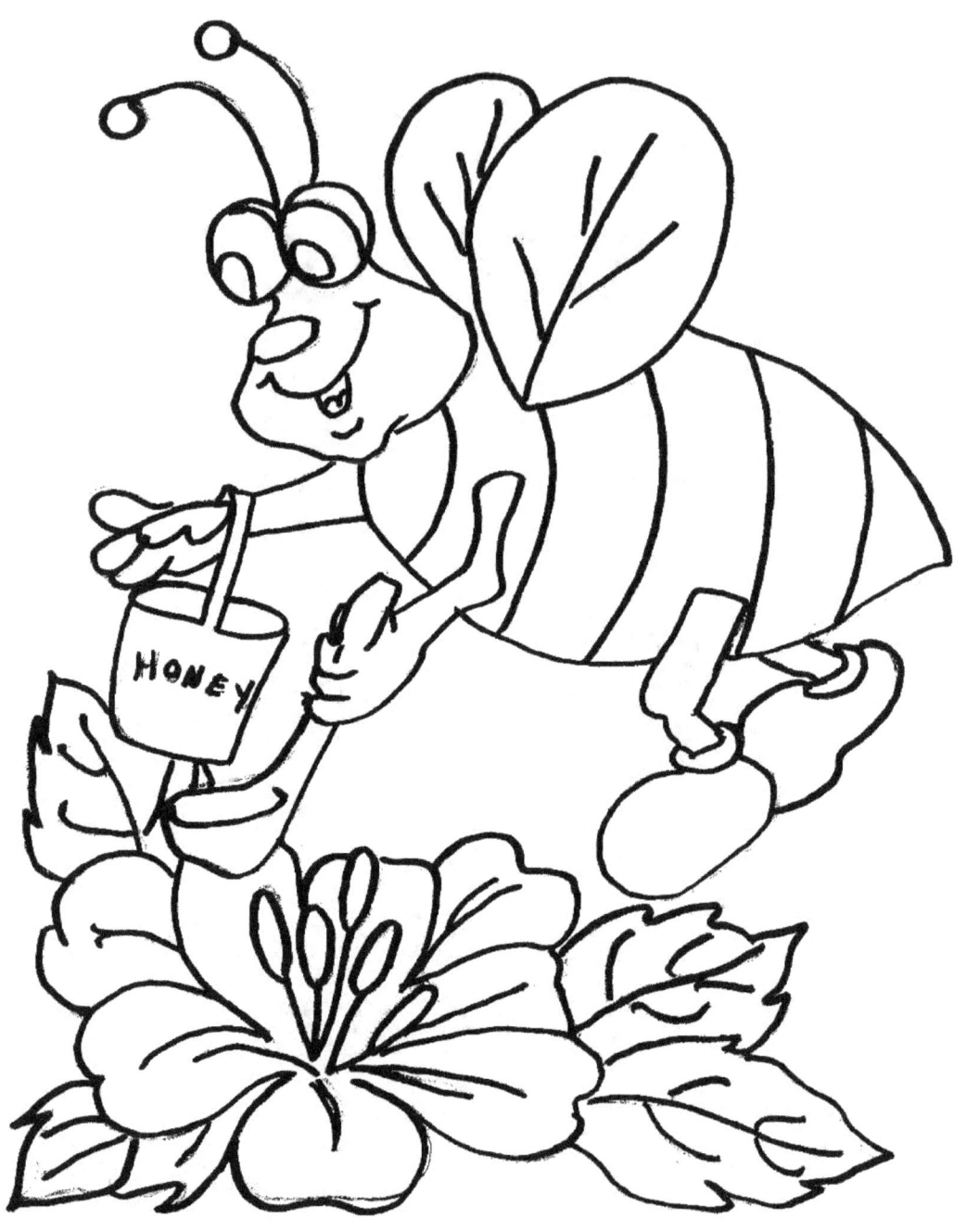

How can honey be used to help us ?

_____

Circle the images showing the healthiest choices.

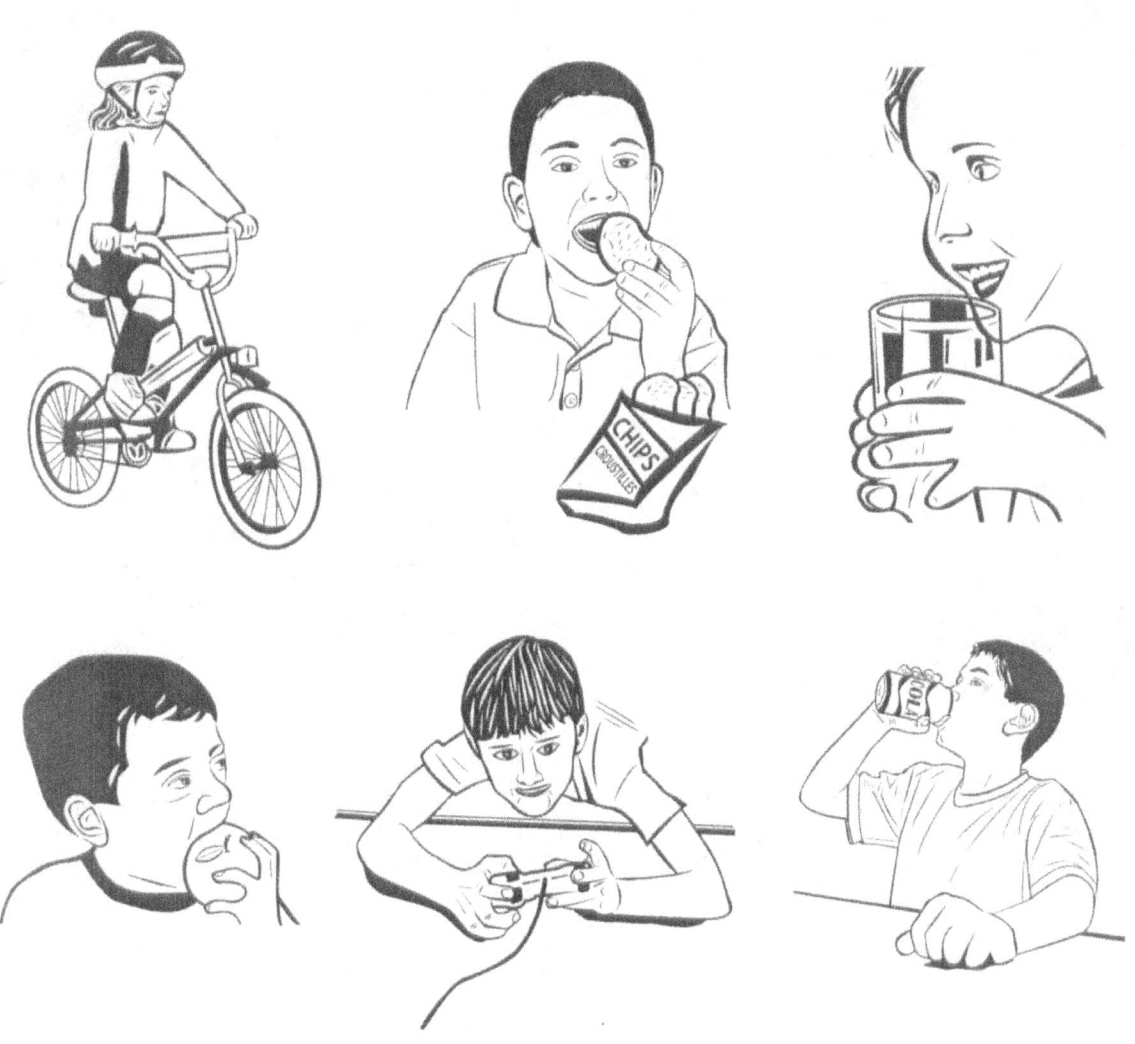

Draw a circle around the most **HEALTHY** activities.

Then, draw your own picture of a way to stay healthy.

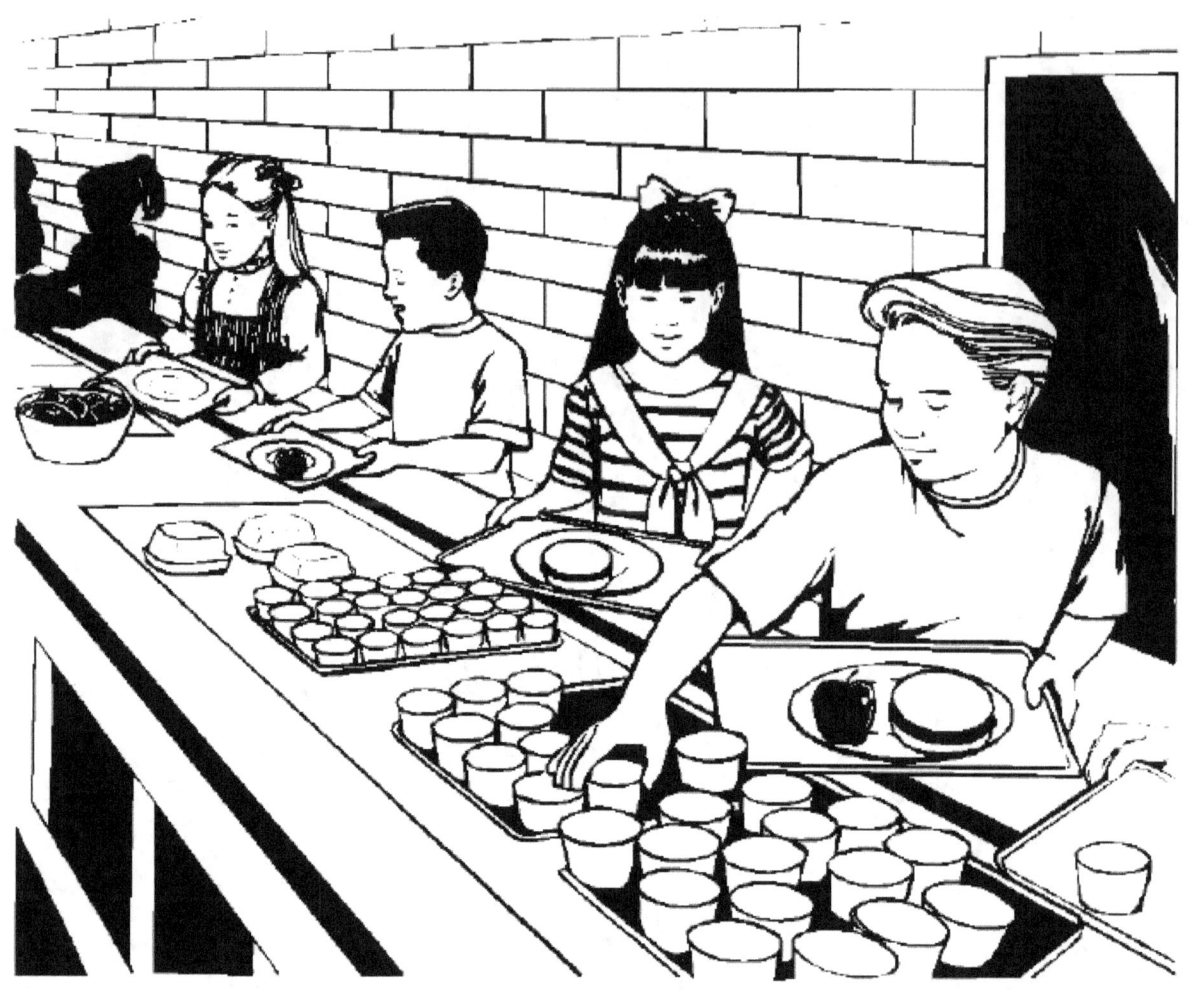

Color this picture. Then choose 4 letters from the alphabet -- and make a list of some healthy things you would like to eat for lunch. The letter should be the first letter of the food that you choose.

Examples: **A**= apple   **E**= egg   **O** = orange juice

_____

_____

_____

DRAW A CIRCLE AROUND THE PICTURES THAT SHOW
ACTIONS THAT ARE <u>**NOT GOOD**</u> FOR GETTING FIT AND
STAYING HEALTHY…. BODY AND MIND --

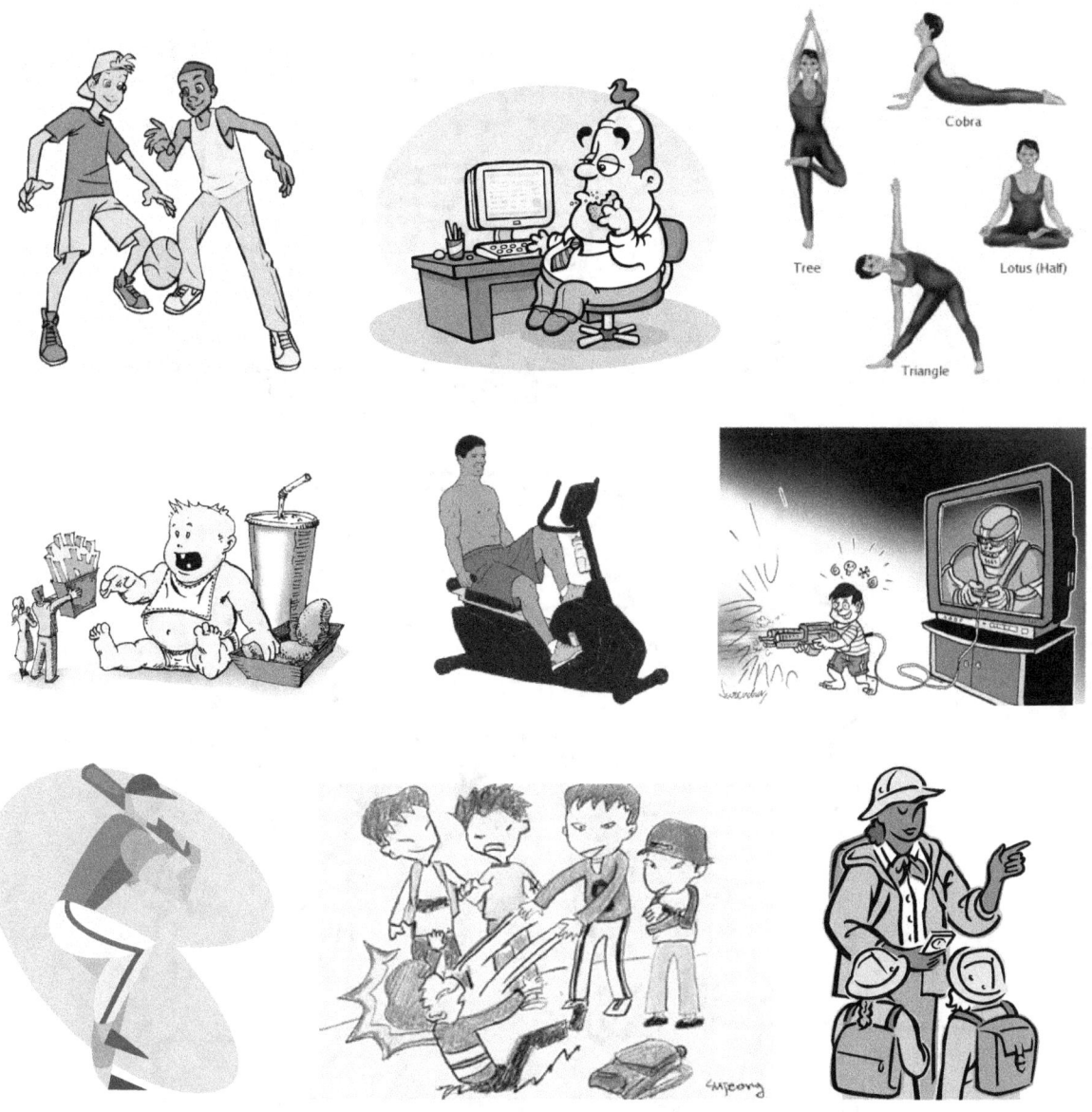

WANT TO STAY IN GOOD HEALTH?   *MOVE!*

How many ways can you think of to get some exercise?

WE NEED LOTS OF **EXERCISE** TO STAY FIT AND HEALTHY

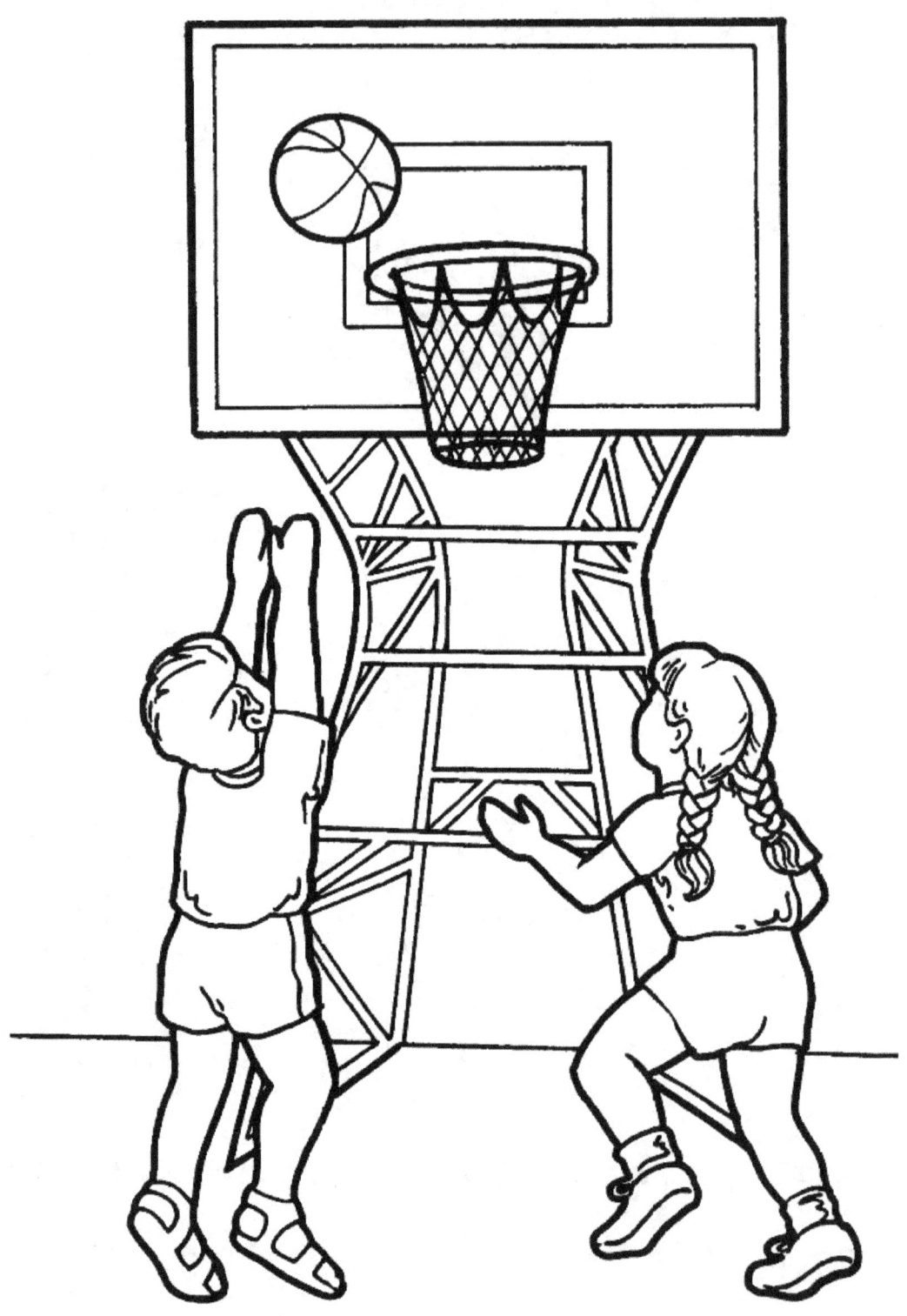

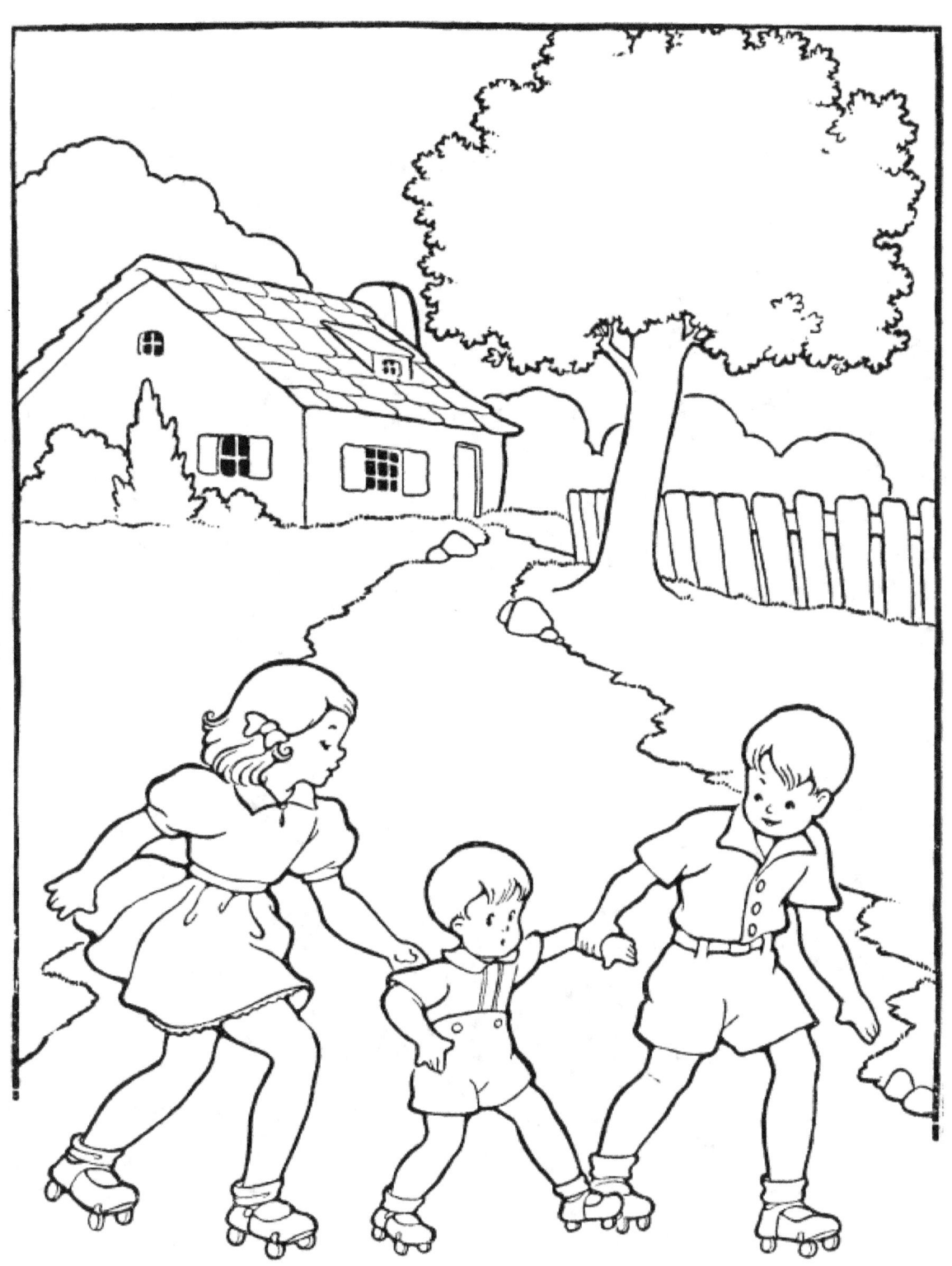

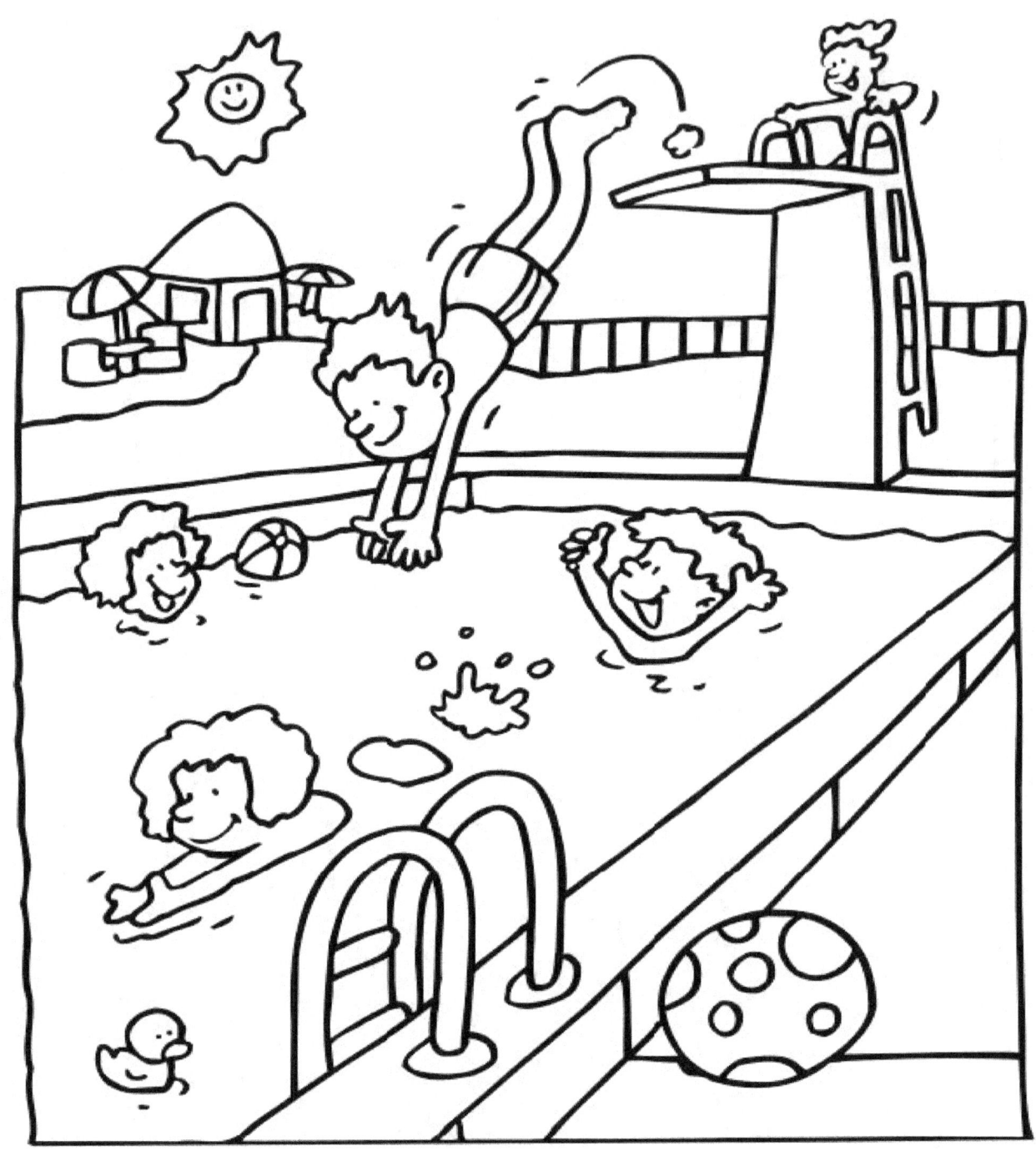

DANCING IS ANOTHER WAY TO GET SOME EXERCISE

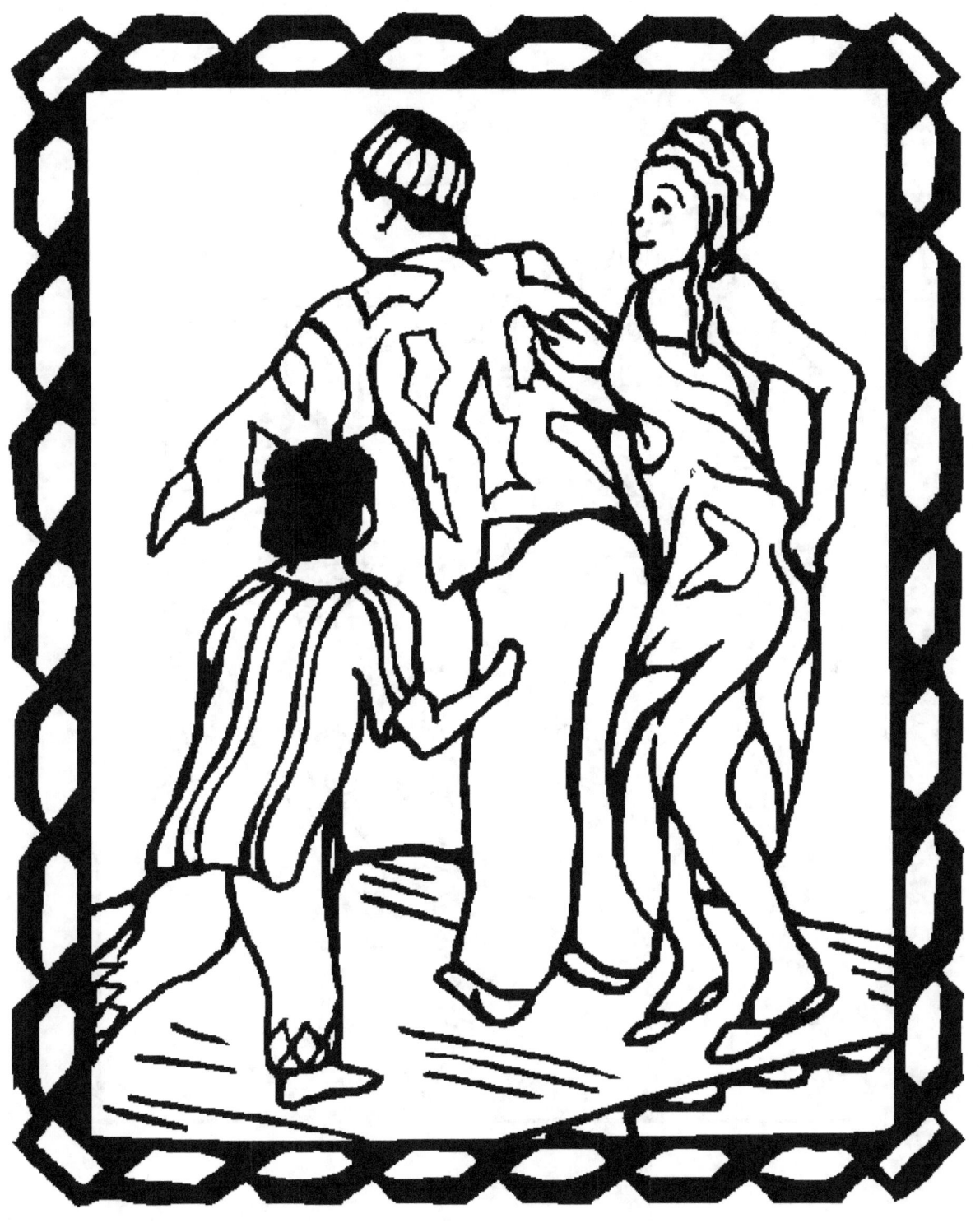

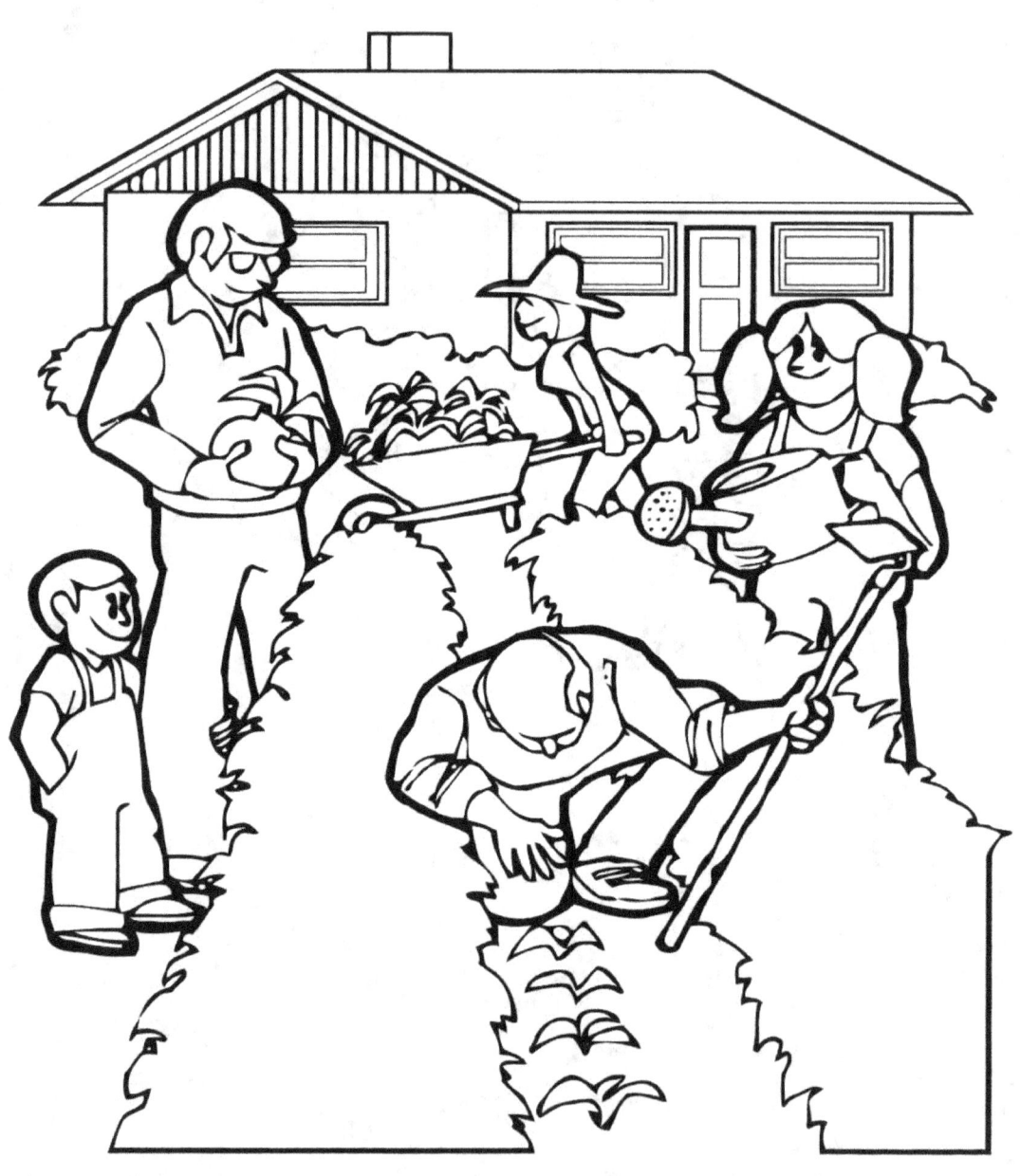

ABOUT

SCIENCE

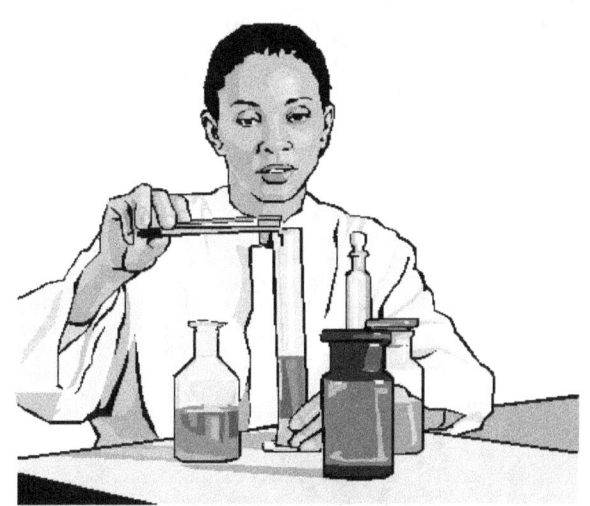

AND

EXPERTS

COLORS FOR OUR HEALTH

ACTIVITY -- **Draw a line from the color to the picture.** Match the color on the left with something that is that color. Then sketch you own picture of something HEALTHY of those colors...so that you will have 2 pictures for each color.

Example -- RED -------------→

Your sketch: apple

YELLOW ------

Your sketch: _____

BLUE ---

Your sketch: _____

BROWN ------

Your sketch _____

WHITE -----

Your sketch: _____

MAKE YOUR OWN HEALTH INFO CARDS...

MAKE CARDS THAT SHOW WHAT EXPERTS, DOCTORS, and NUTRITIONISTS SAY ABOUT THE ITEMS THAT YOU HAVE MATCHED WITH THE COLORS.

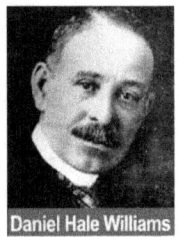
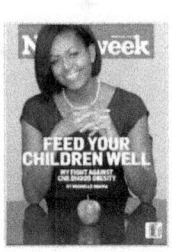
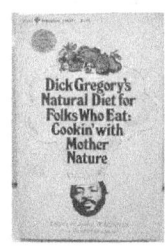
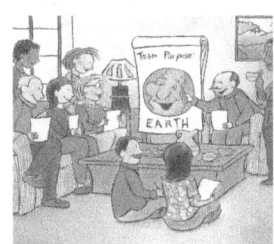
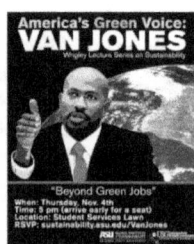

Dr. George Washington Carver made 300 products for peanuts and 100 from potatoes.

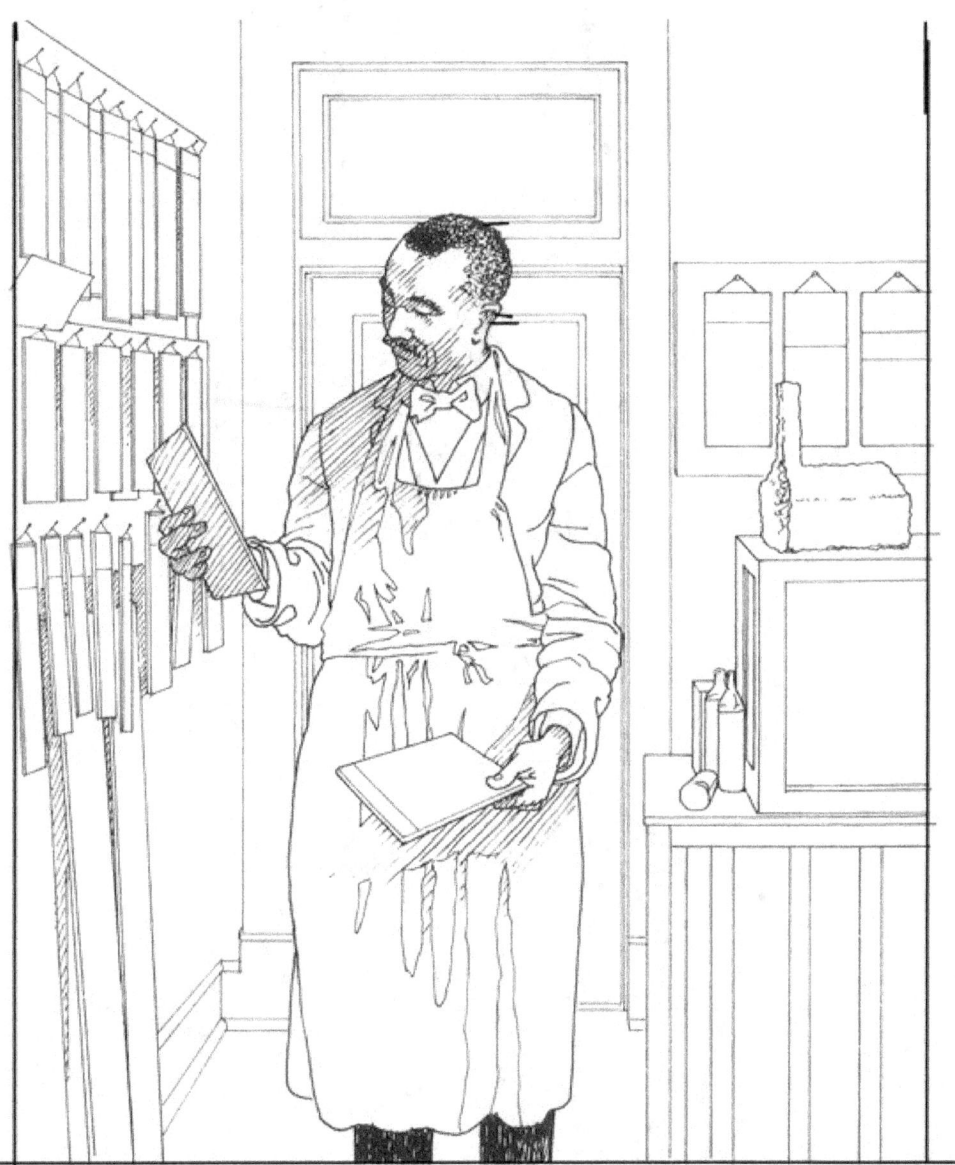

GEORGE WASHINGTON CARVER (1864–1943). Botanist. Born into slavery, Carver obtained a high-school education in his twenties and received a degree in agricultural science in 1894. He followed it with a master's in 1896, the year in which he went to Alabama to head the department of agricultural science at the Tuskegee Institute. Carver held that the racial situation would be corrected through education rather than political action, and saw agriculture as a means of bettering the condition of rural African-Americans. He urged the cultivation of legumes, most notably the soybean and peanut, for restoring the fertility of soil that had been exhausted by years devoted to the growth of cotton. In doing this he revolutionized the agriculture of the South.

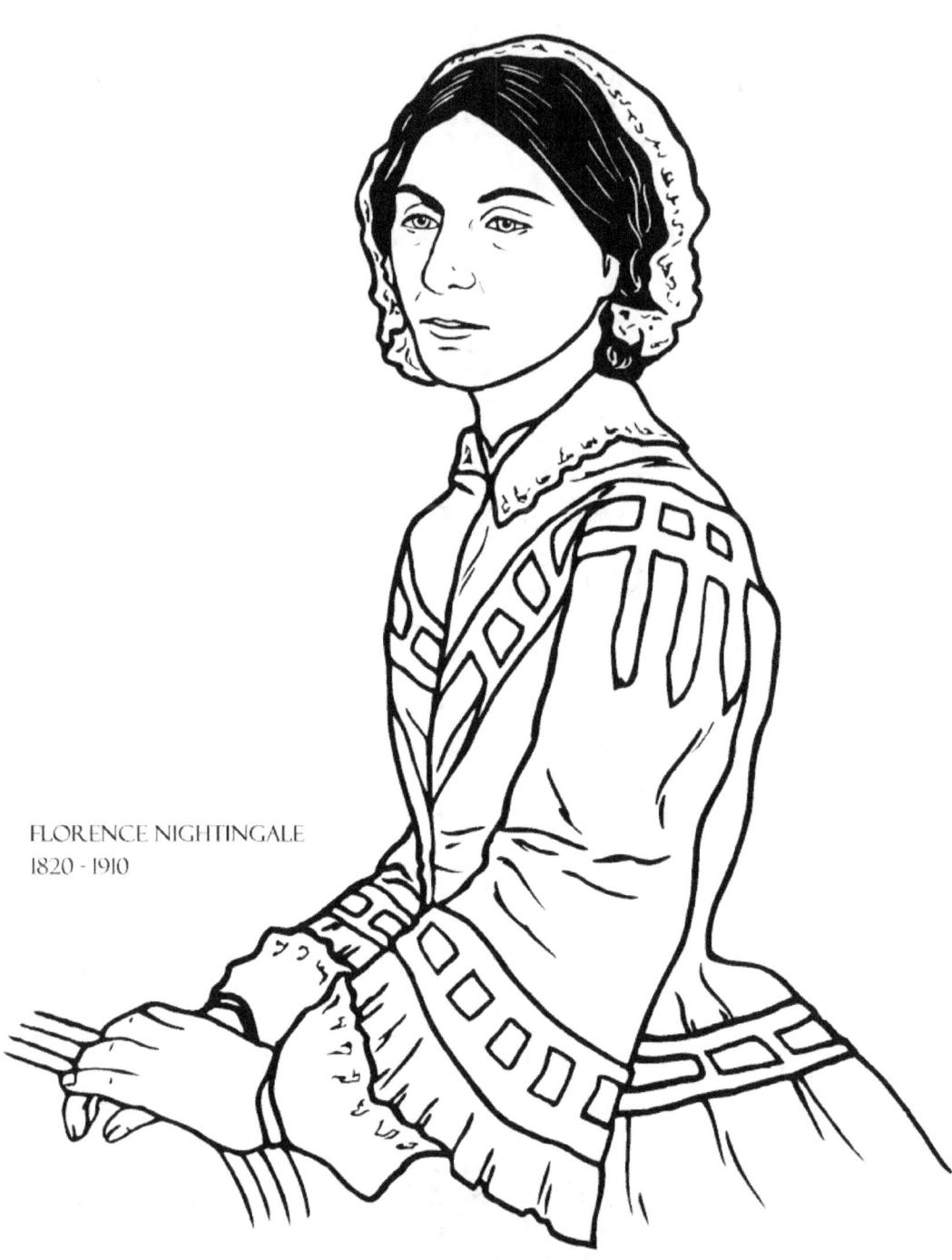

FLORENCE NIGHTINGALE
1820 - 1910

FLORENCE NIGHTINGALE was a celebrated English nurse, writer and statistician. She came to prominence for her pioneering work in nursing during the <u>Crimean War</u>, where she tended to wounded soldiers. She was dubbed *"The Lady with the Lamp"* after her habit of making rounds at night. She established her own Nursing School in 1860 in London.

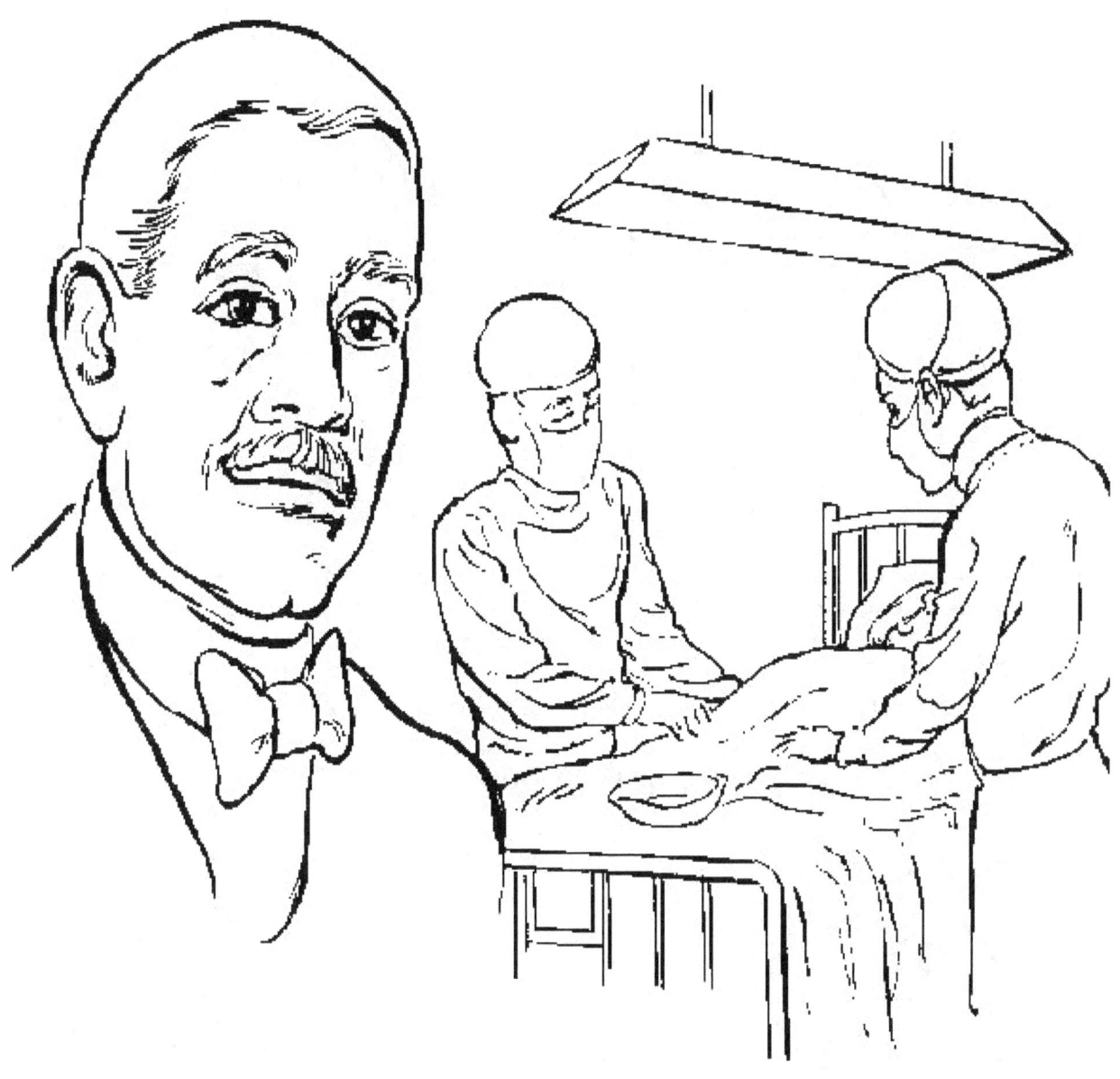

Dr. Daniel Hale Williams

(cardiologist who performed the first successful heart surgery)

Rene *"Cancer Nurse"* Caisse 1888-1978

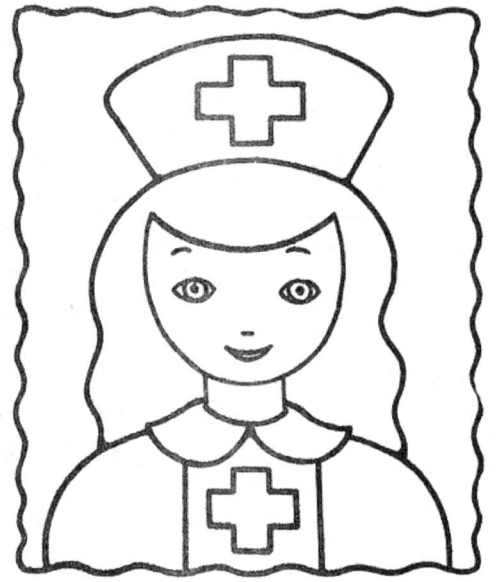

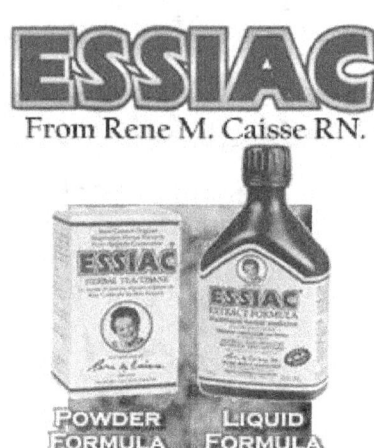

Rene Caisse suffered with breast CANCER, but had no money and no Health Insurance. An old Indian taught her how to make a special herb tea, which amazingly cured her cancer. After that she devoted her life to thousands of terminally ill cancer patients using her **Essiac** formula. The "cancer curing" formula originated from an old Indian herbal TEA formula, that she obtained from a patient in 1922.

CLARA BARTON FOUNDED THE RED CROSS

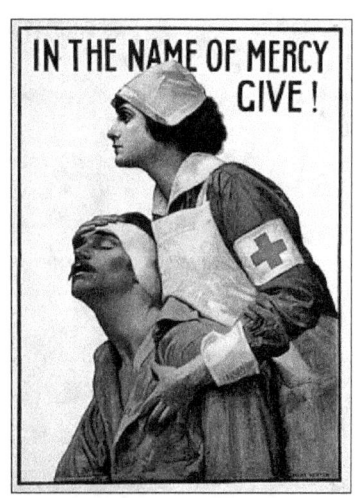

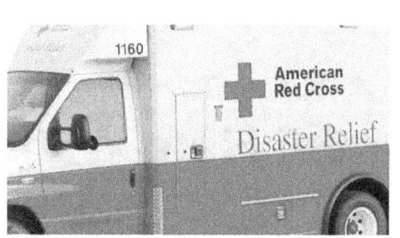

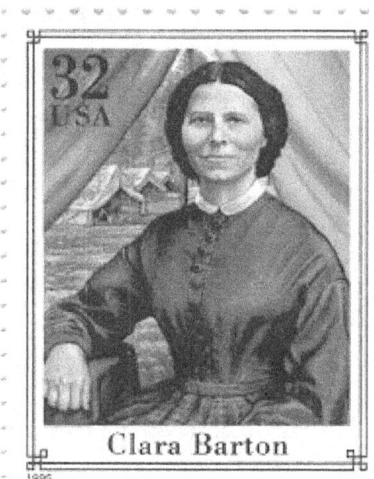

Clara Barton

THE MORE WE KNOW ABOUT OUR BODIES, THE BETTER WE
CAN TAKE CARE OF OURSELVES.

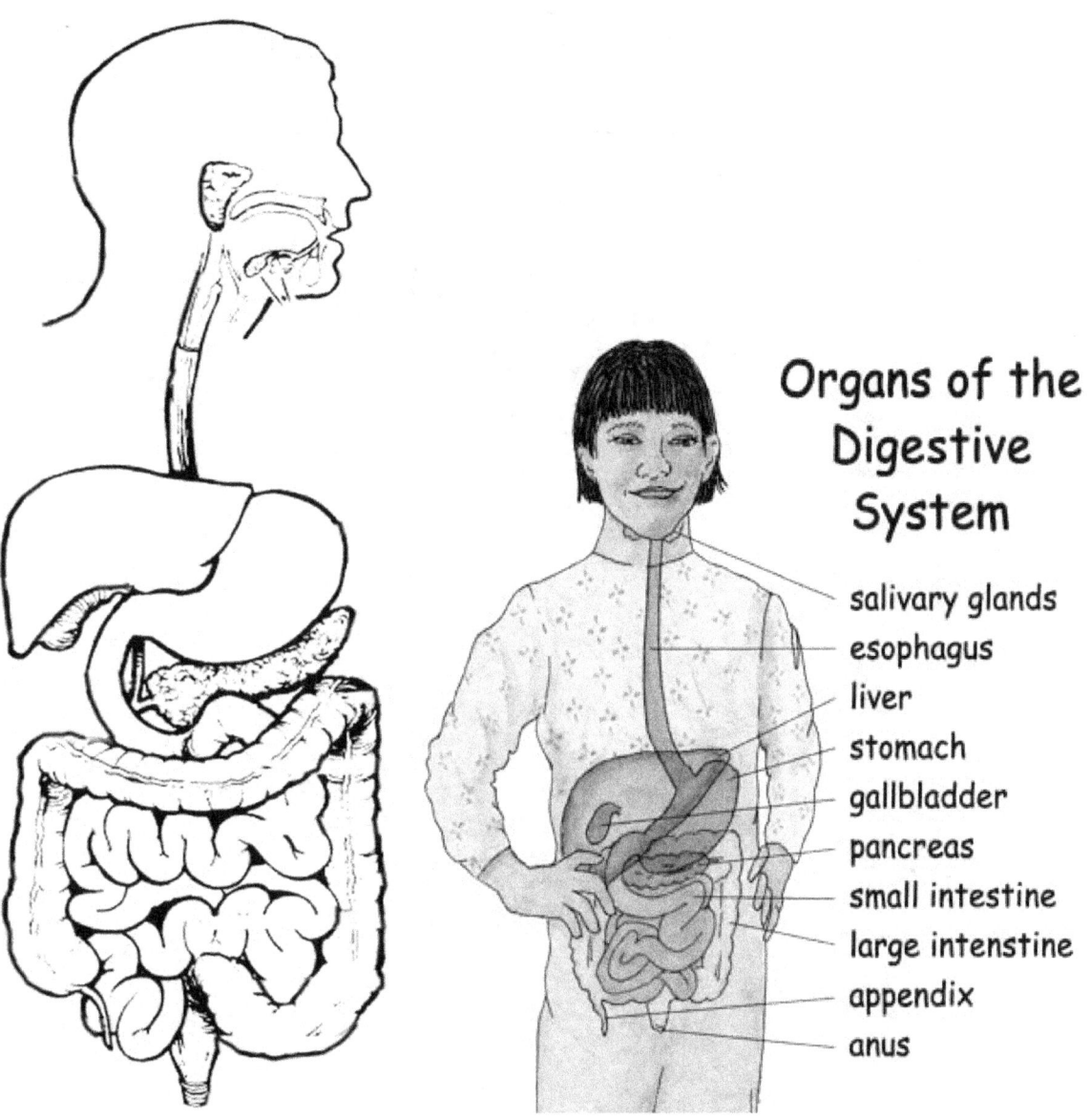

Organs of the
Digestive
System

salivary glands
esophagus
liver
stomach
gallbladder
pancreas
small intestine
large intenstine
appendix
anus

HARMFUL TO THE DIGESTIVE SYSTEM = Too much soda pop, sugars, alcohol, chemicals.

NAME A FOOD OR DRINK THAT IS <u>DIFFICULT</u> TO DIGEST –

_____

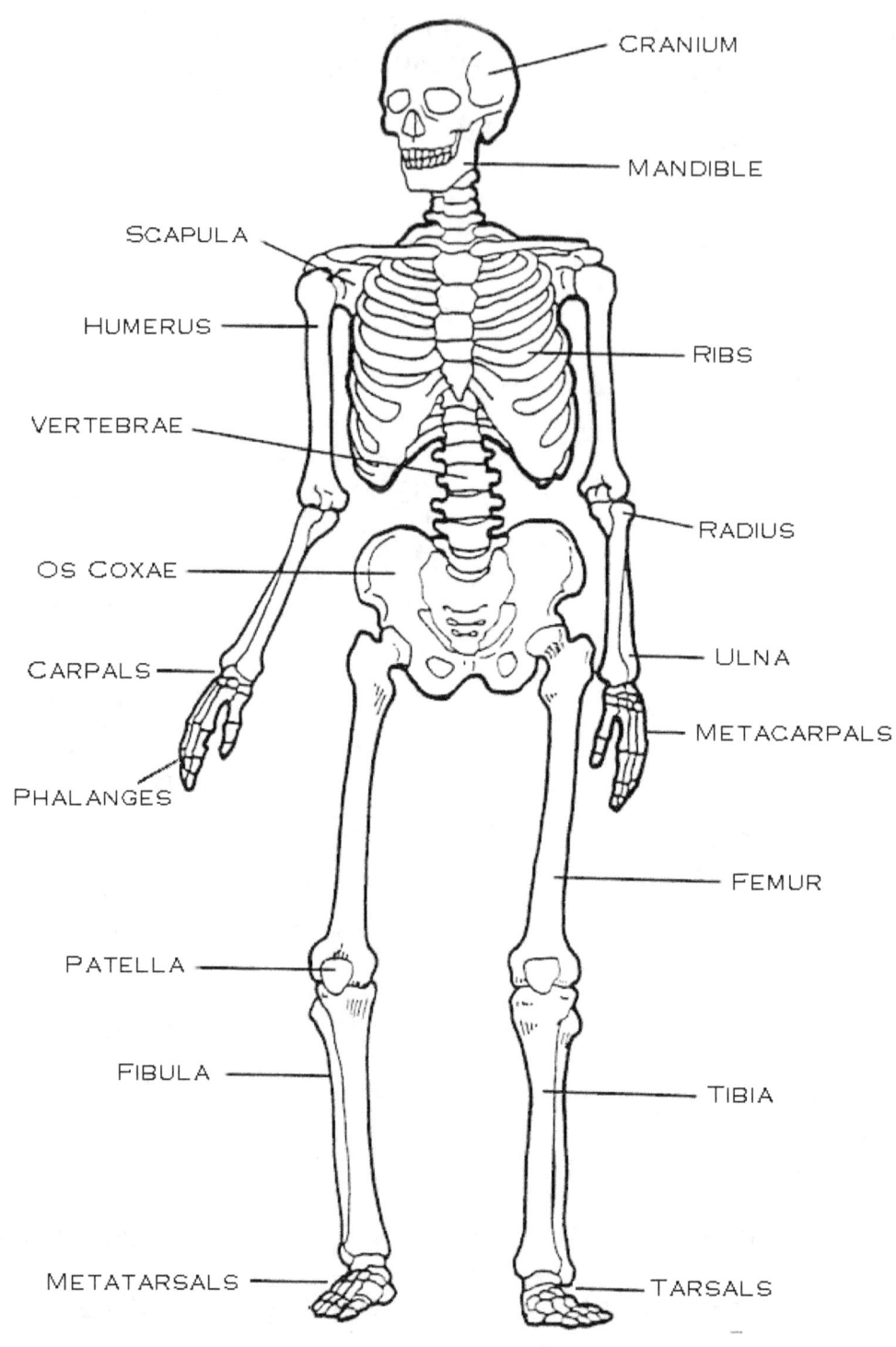

CRANIUM

MANDIBLE

SCAPULA

HUMERUS

RIBS

VERTEBRAE

RADIUS

OS COXAE

ULNA

CARPALS

METACARPALS

PHALANGES

FEMUR

PATELLA

FIBULA

TIBIA

METATARSALS

TARSALS

Our bones need minerals to grow and stay strong.

ABOUT

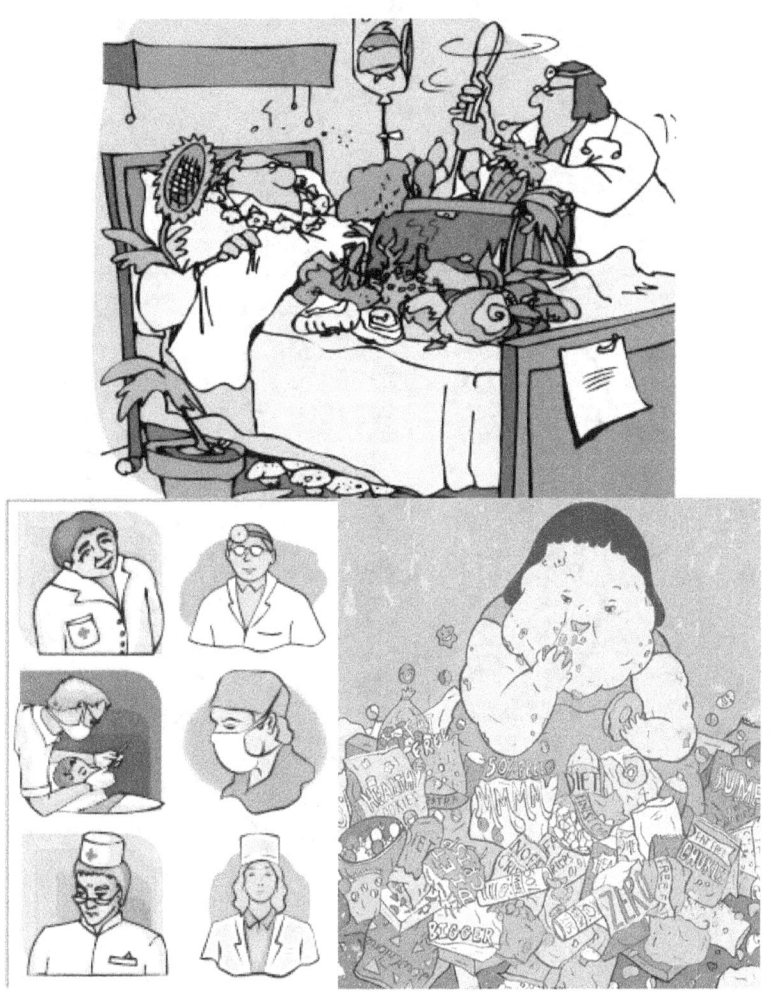

HEALING

SICKNESS

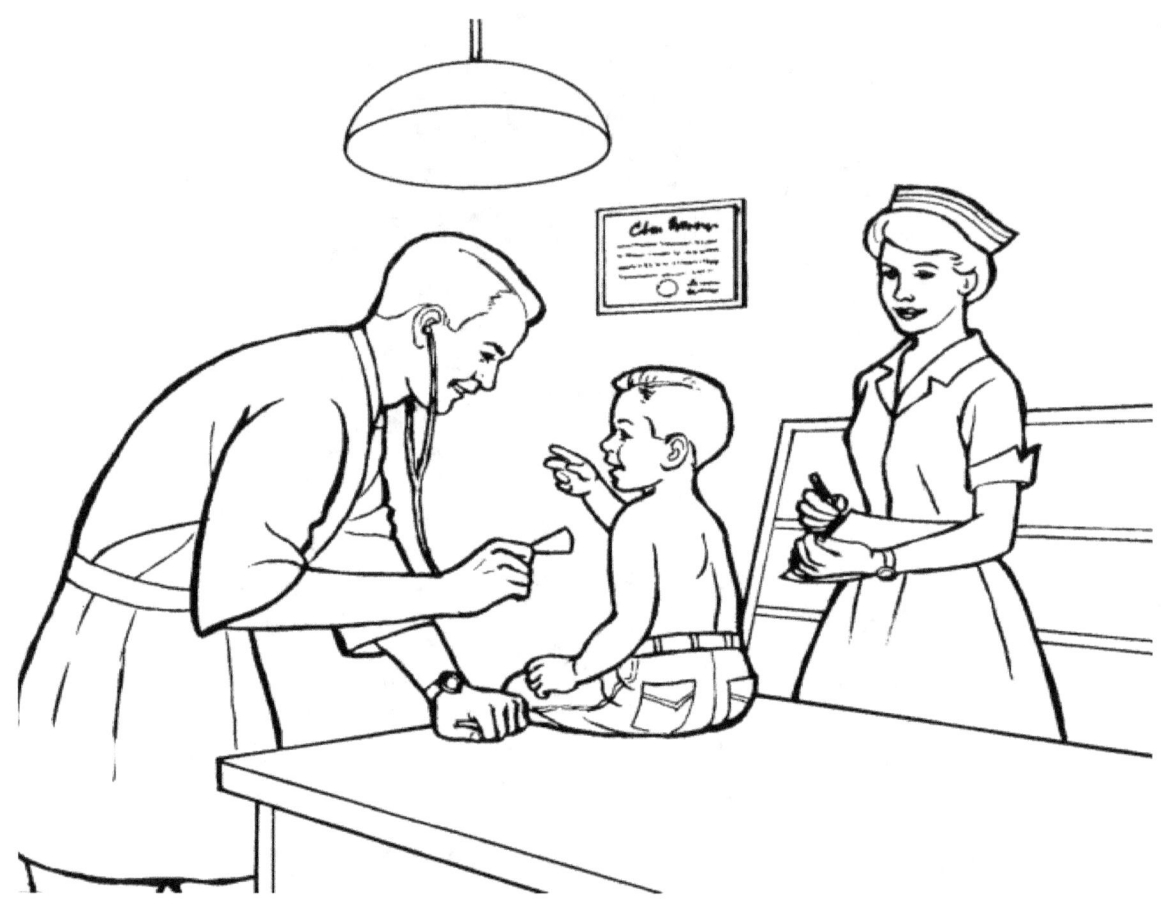

A Doctor makes sure we are heathy

And if you get sick, you may
need to see your doctor.

What's Wrong?

My name is _____

What's wrong?

I have a cough

I have

a runny nose   a cough   a sore throat
a headache   a cold   a fever

Get Well Soon!

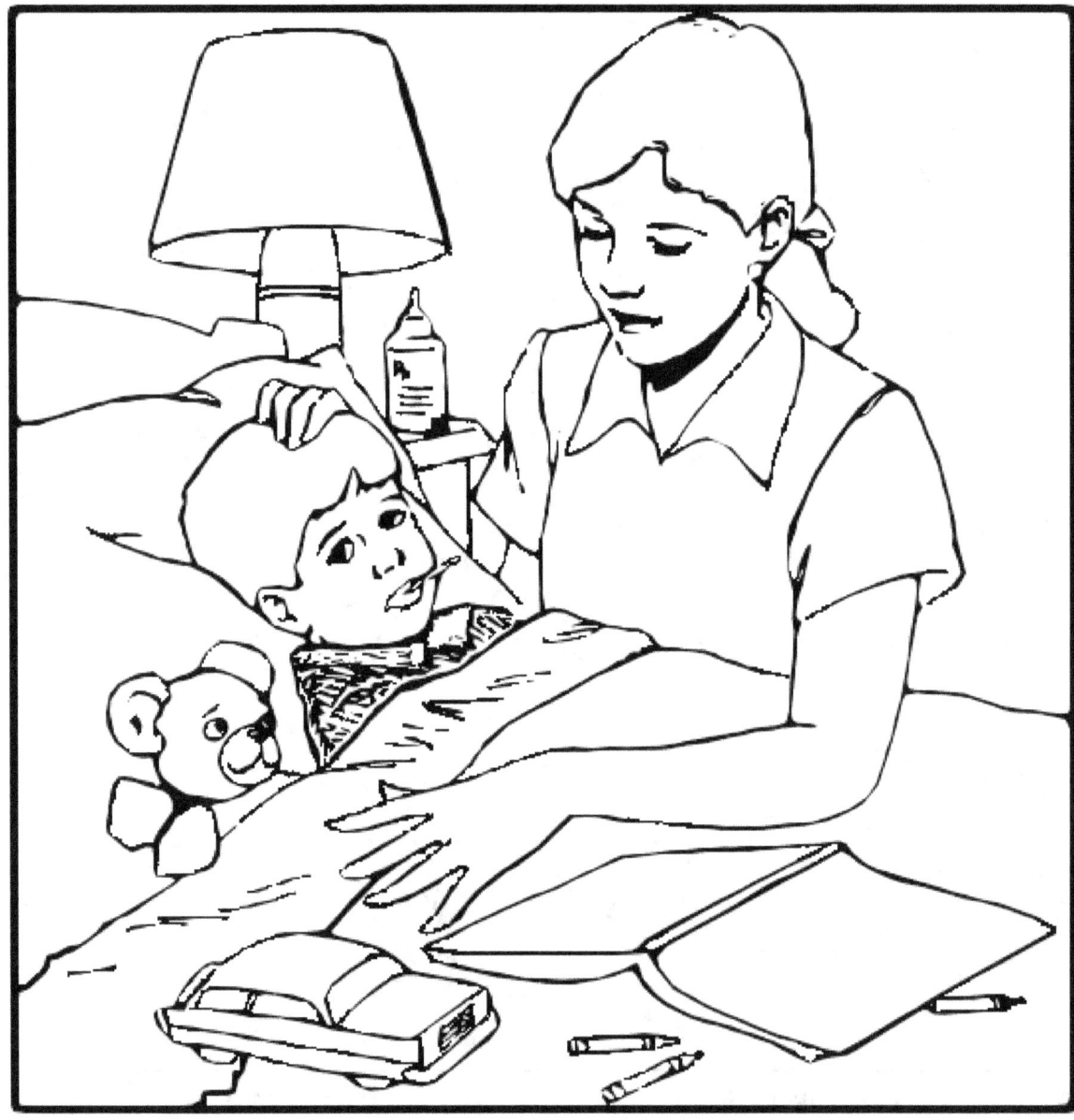

If you get sick, get lots of rest and drink lots of liquids – like water and juices.

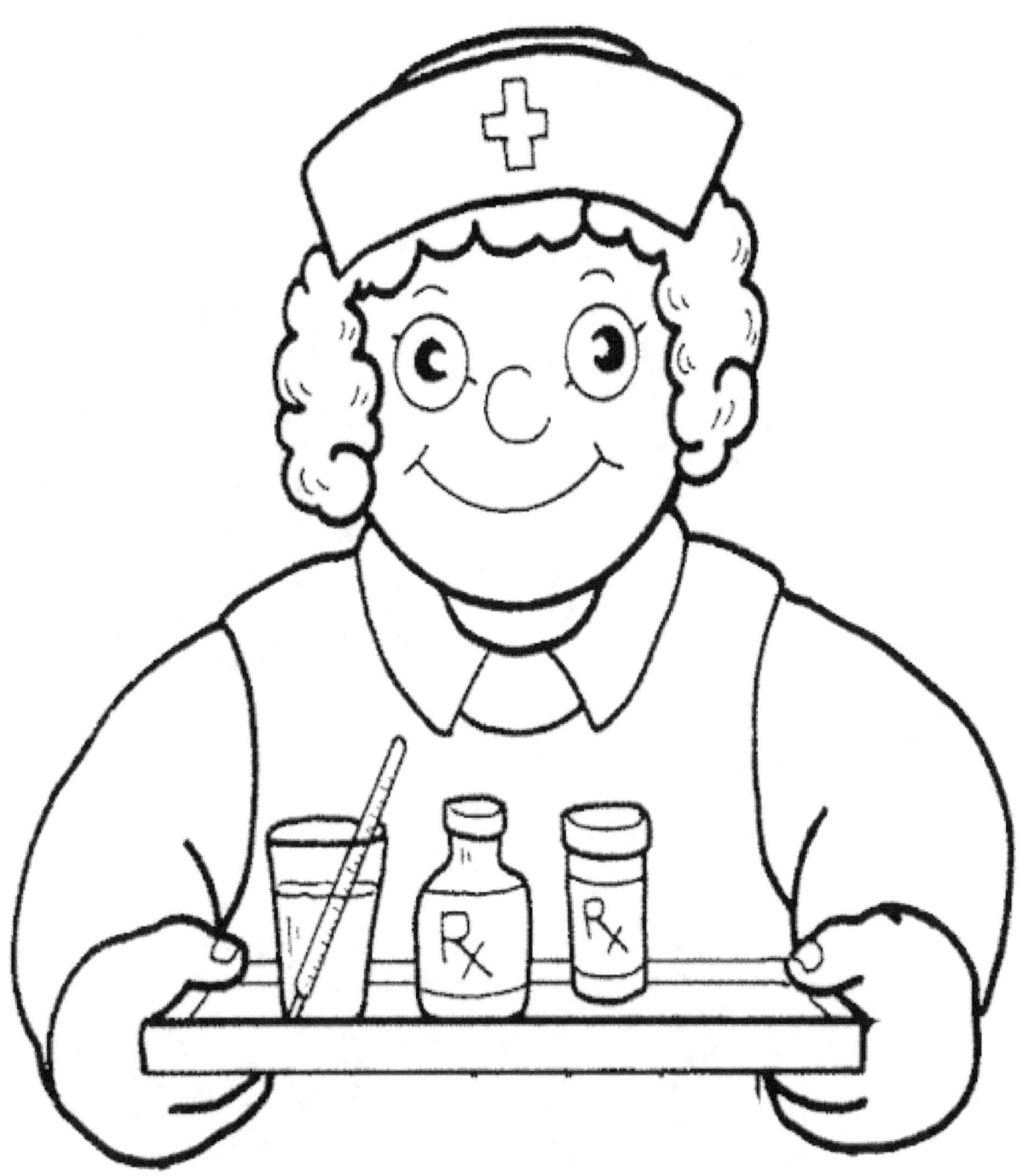

Name one duty of a NURSE _____

THERE ARE MANY METHODS WE CAN USE TO GET AND STAY WELL.

Can you name what these people do to help improve health?

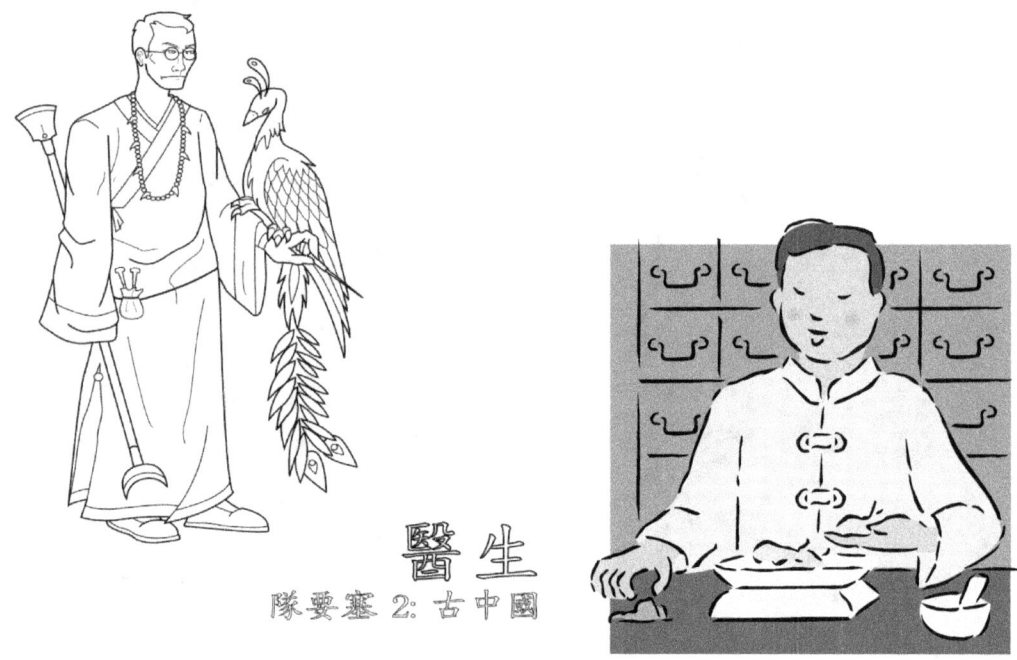

醫生

隊要塞 2: 古中國

Describe: _____

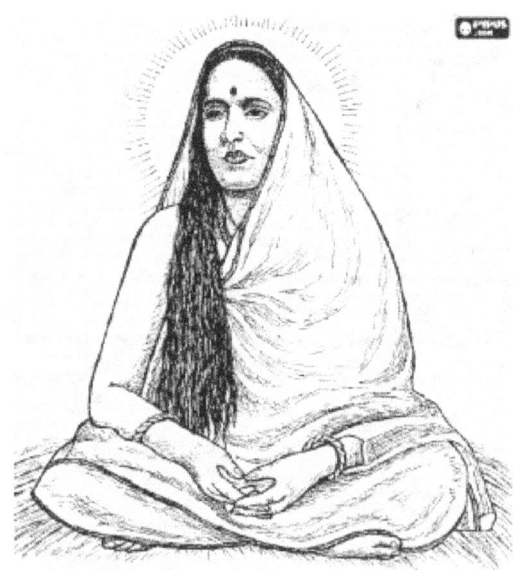

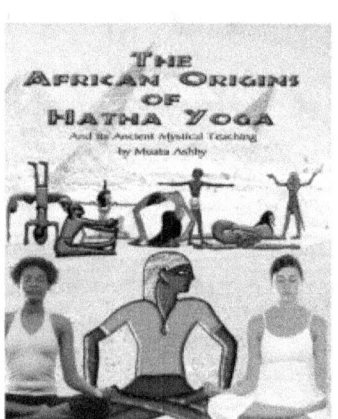

Describe: _____

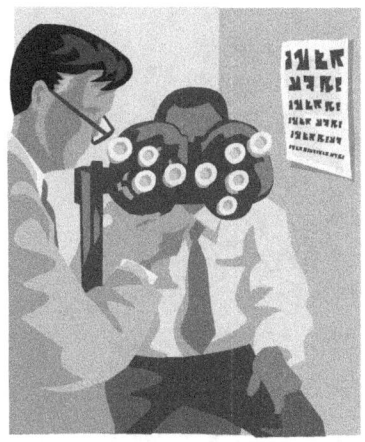 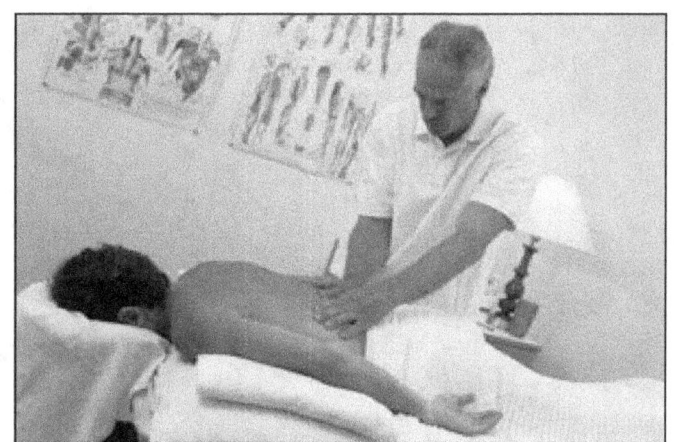

Describe _____

_____

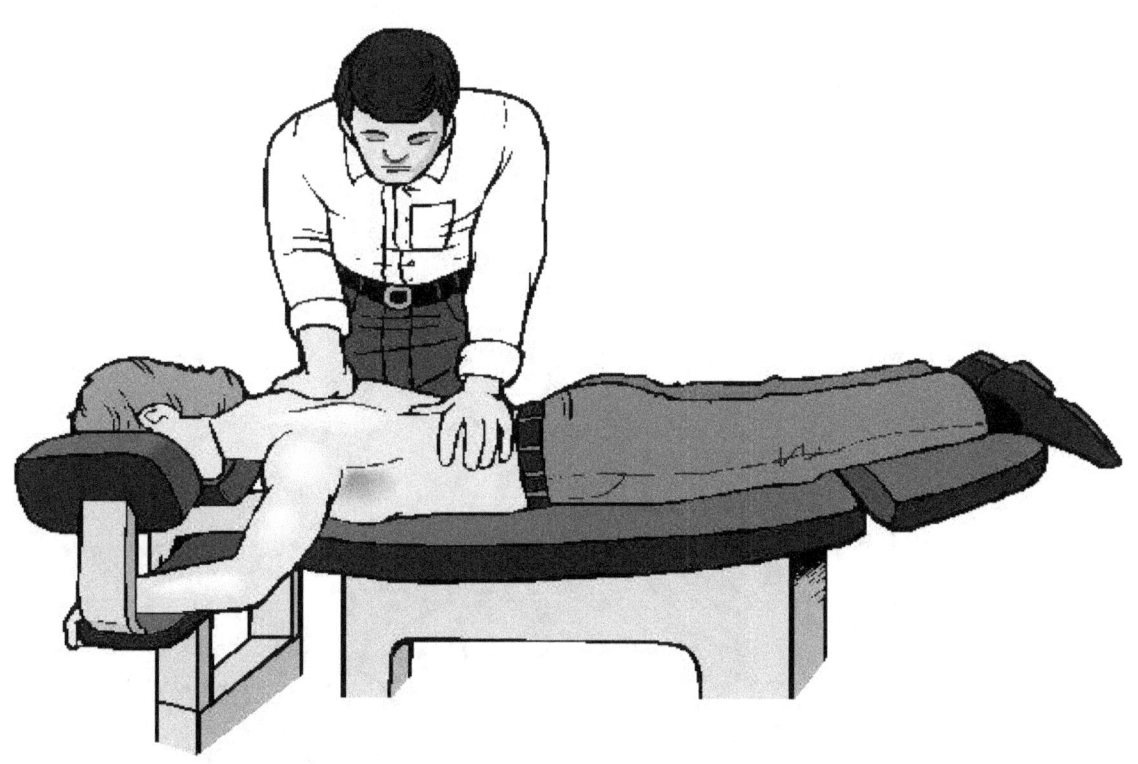

This **Chiropractor** is doing what? _____

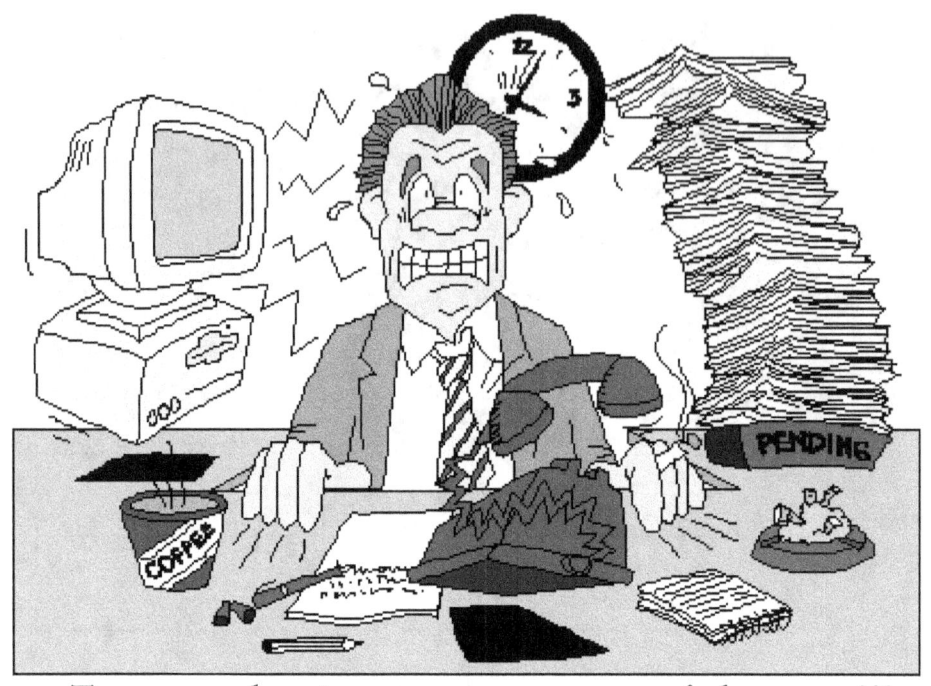

Too much **stress** can cause sickness !!!

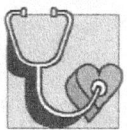

DO YOU WANT TO HAVE MORE ENERGY?
ARE YOU TRYING TO LOSE WEIGHT?
WOULD YOU LIKE TO FEEL BETTER MENTALLY?

WOULD YOU LIKE TO HAVE MORE ENERGY & VITALITY?

DID YOU KNOW? ....without proper nutrition, you will get sick

....your body will not be able to function properly.

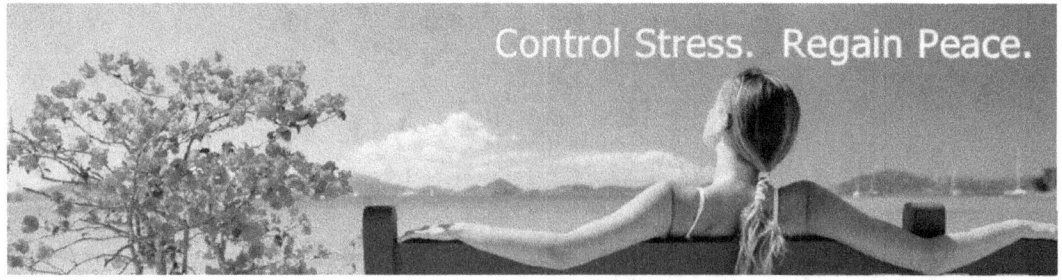

Control Stress. Regain Peace.

ABOUT NATURE

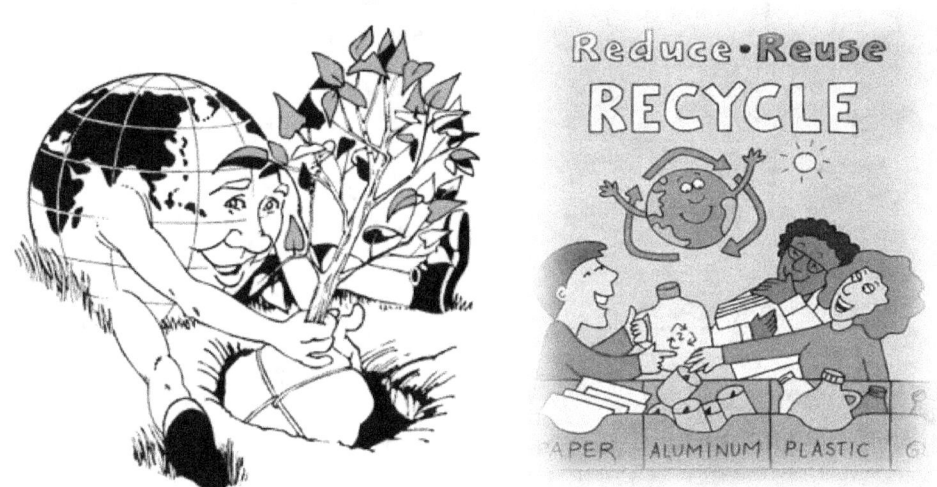

AND
THE EARTH

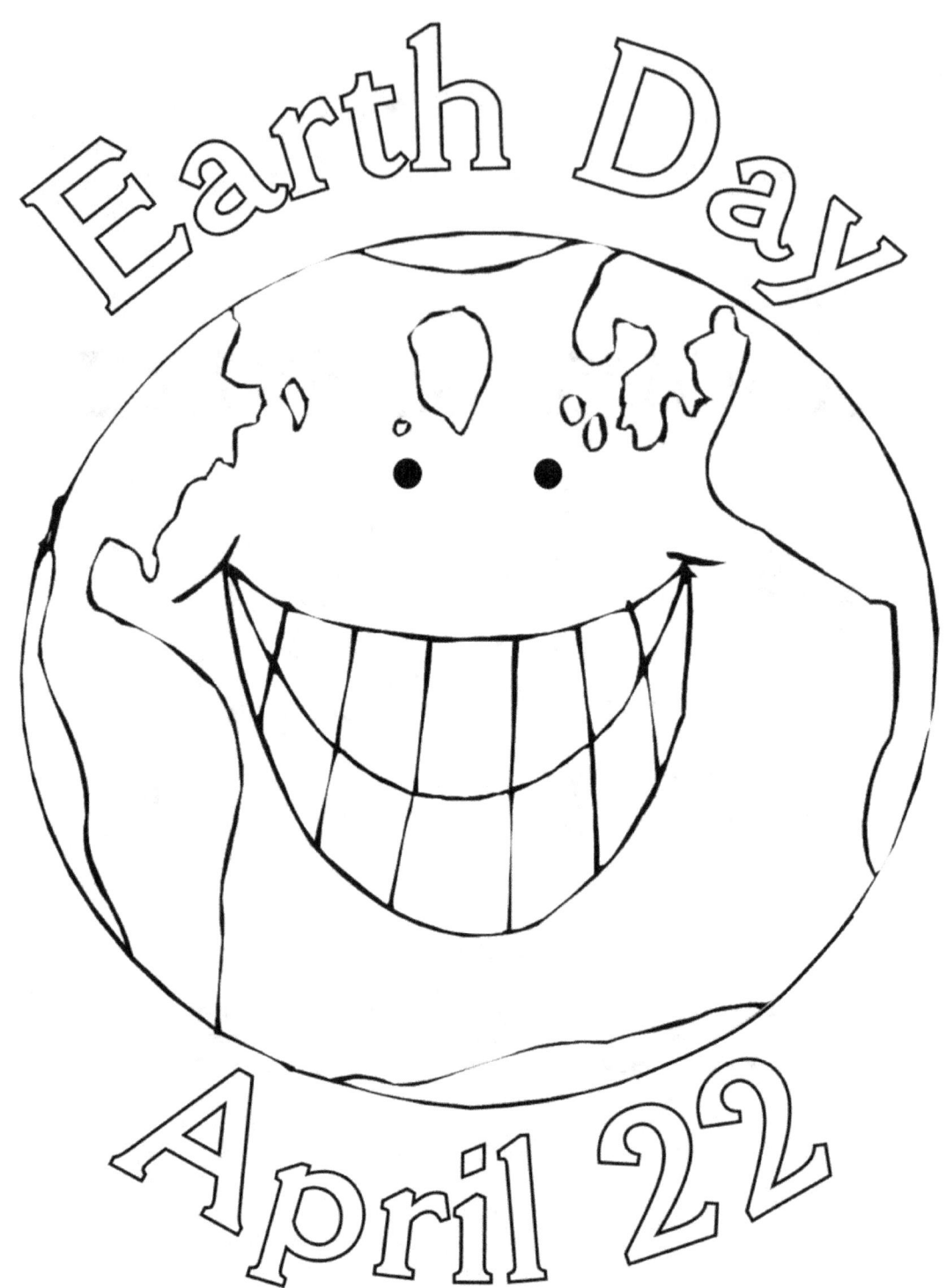

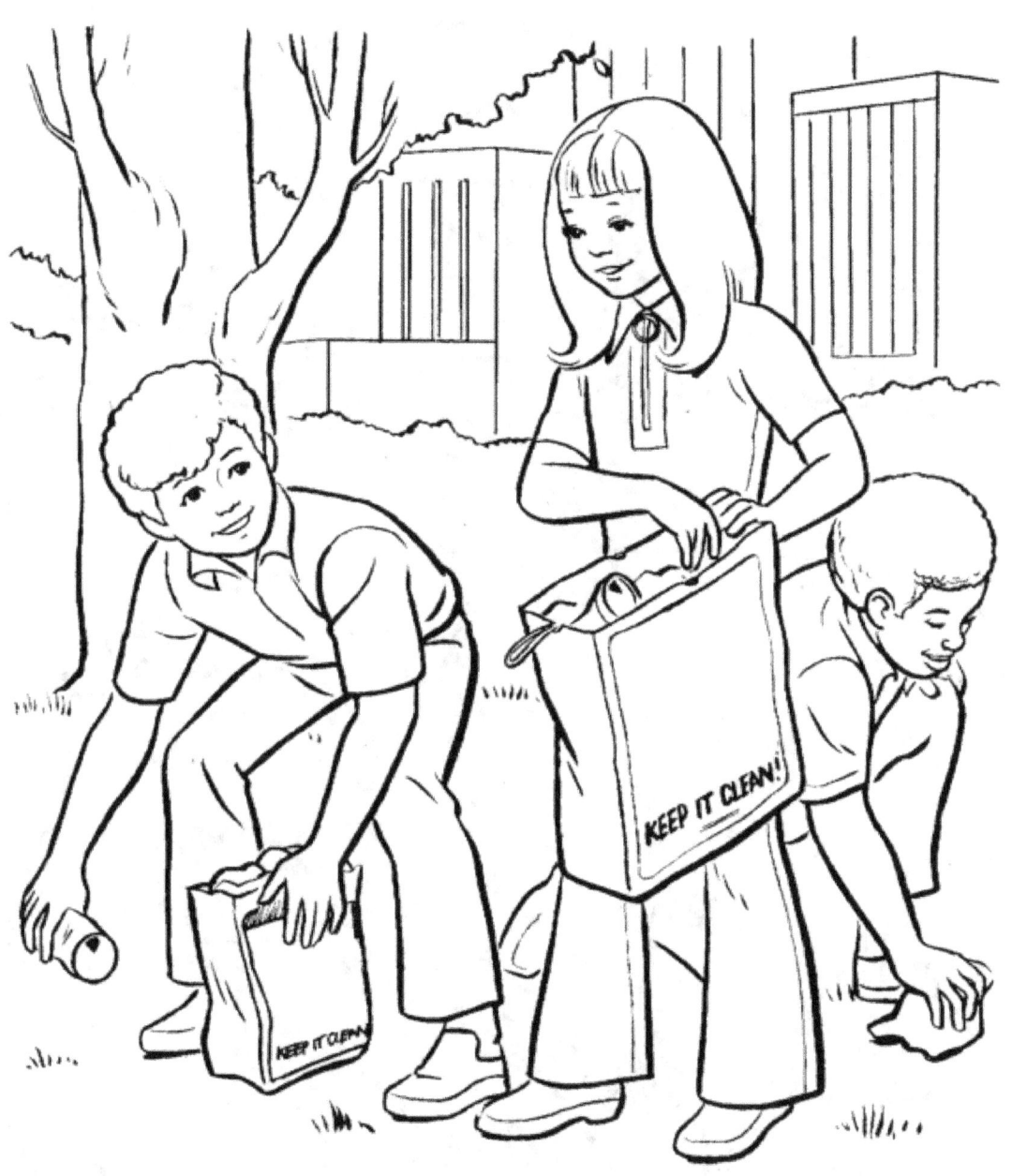

"JOIN THE CLEAN-UP TEAM. HELP KEEP OUR LAND CLEAN."

We can learn about food and health – while
enjoying Nature by gardening...

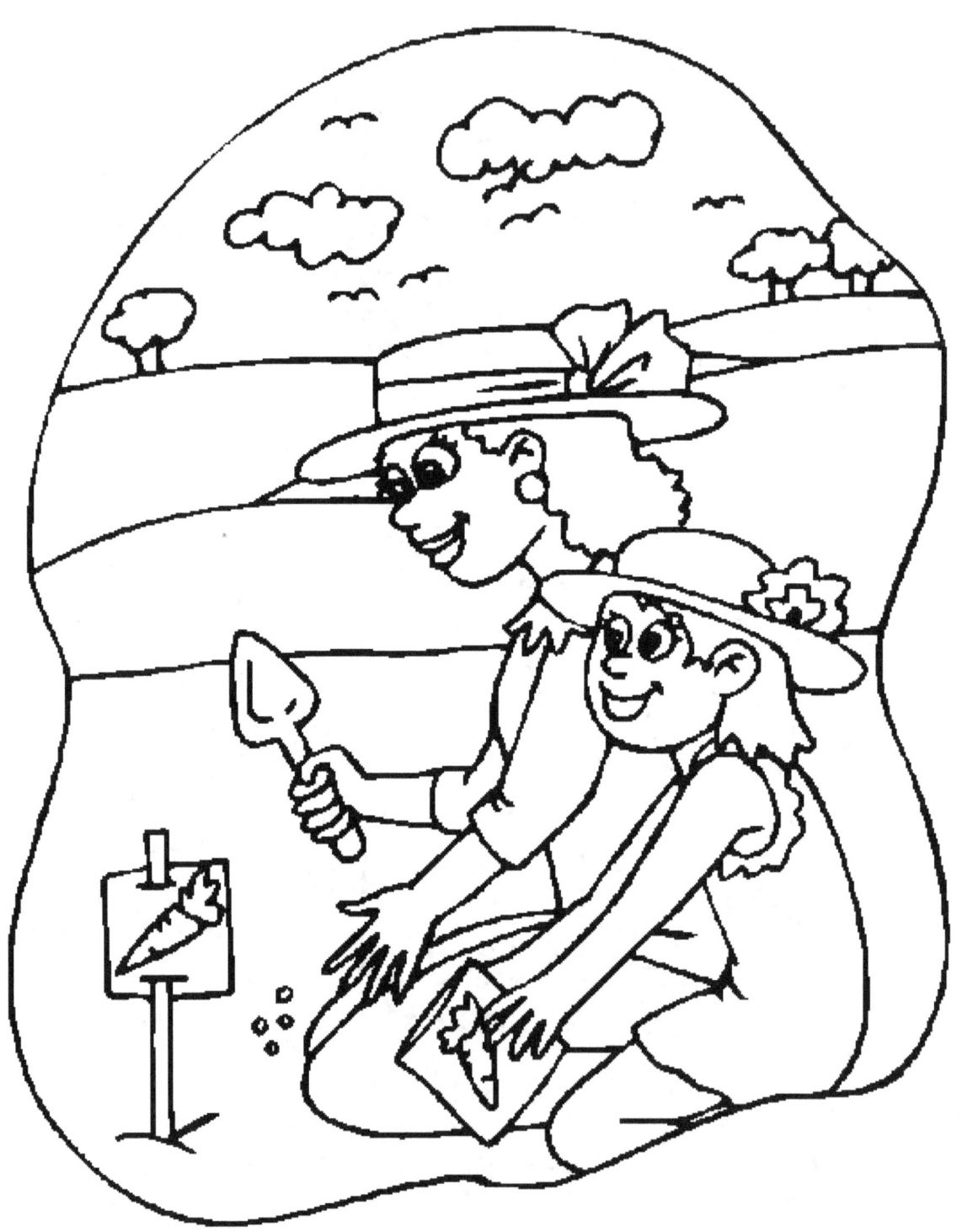

Earth offers many gifts...

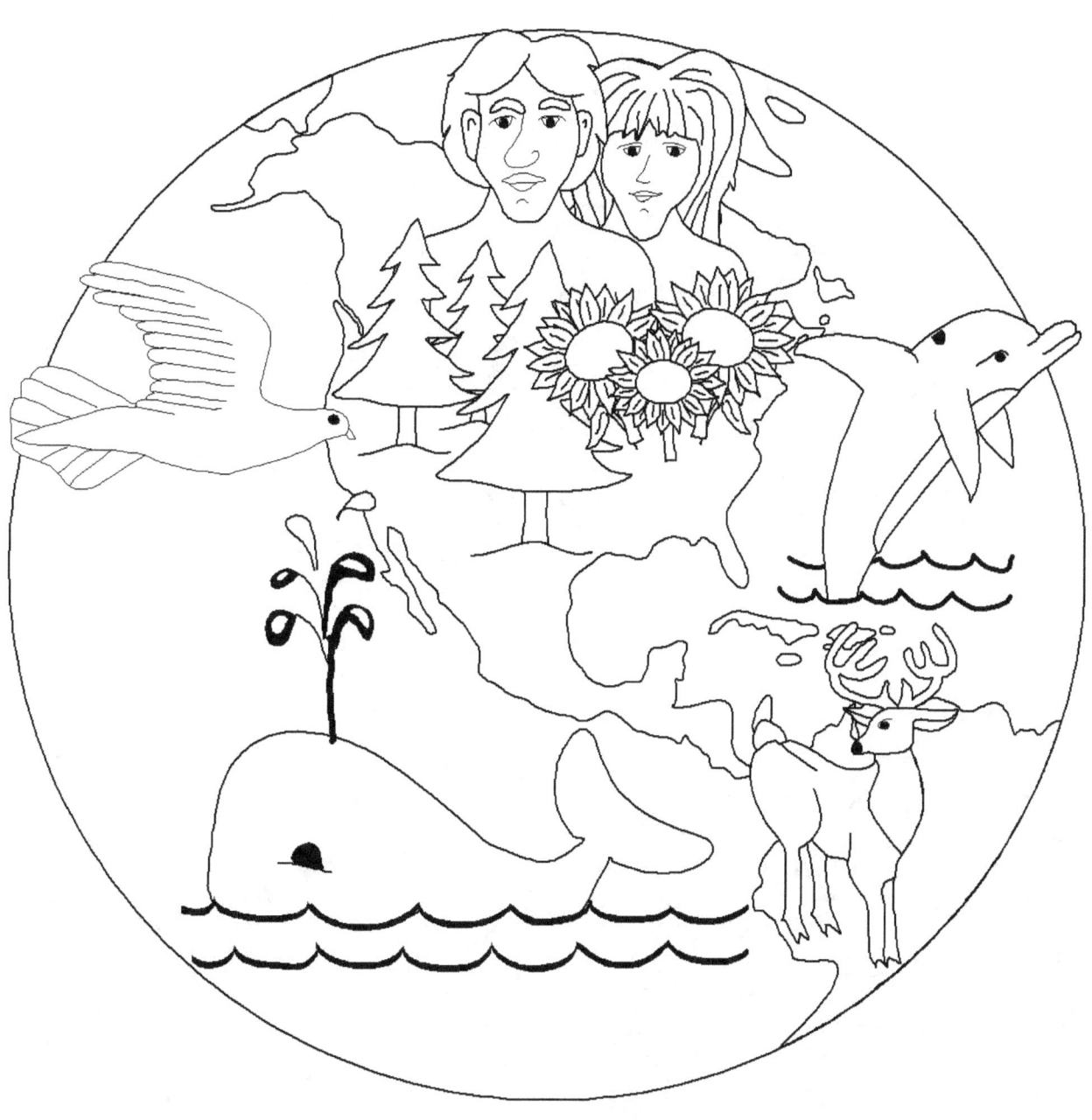

GET **OUTSIDE** – ENJOY **NATURE** MORE OFTEN

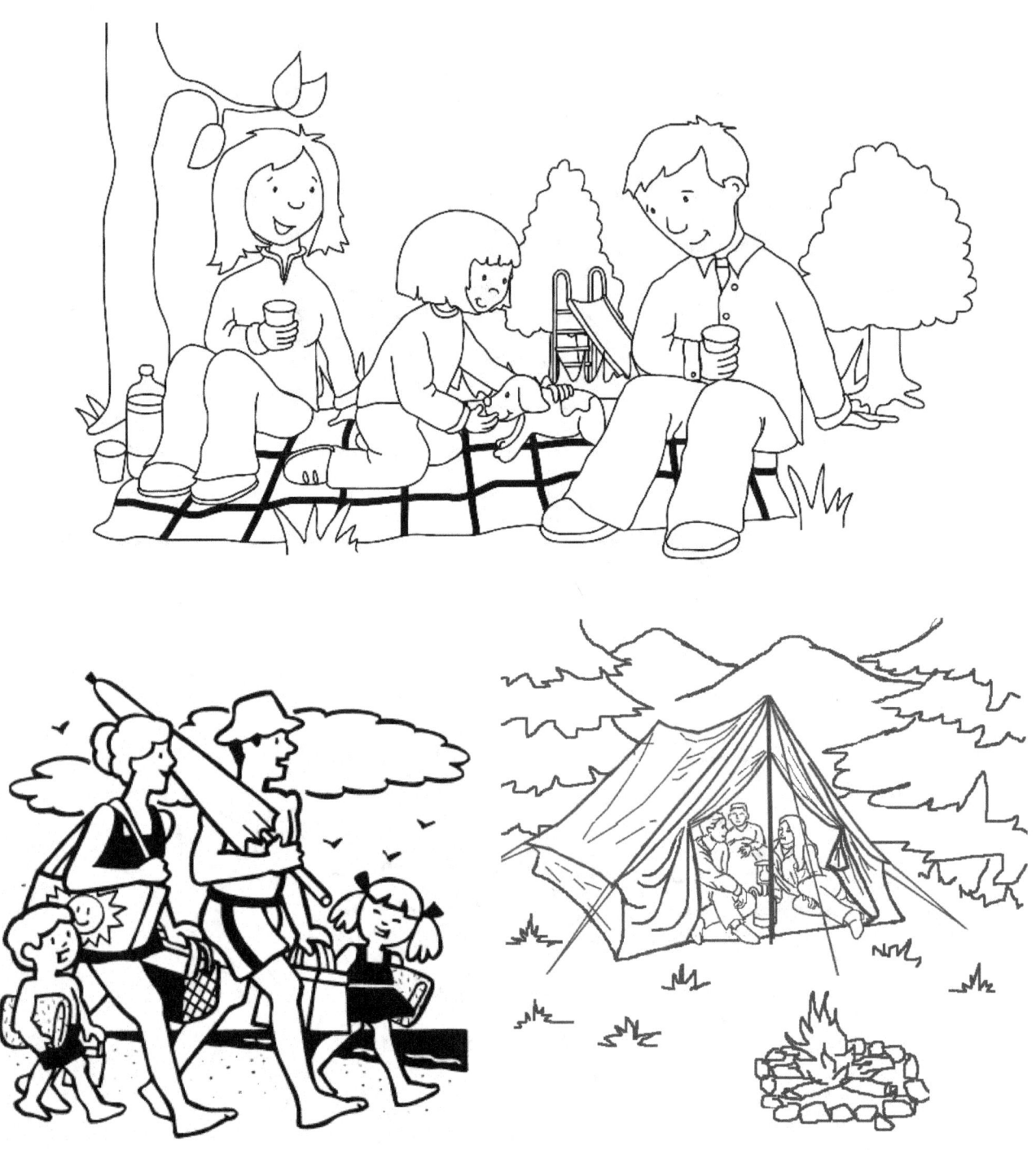

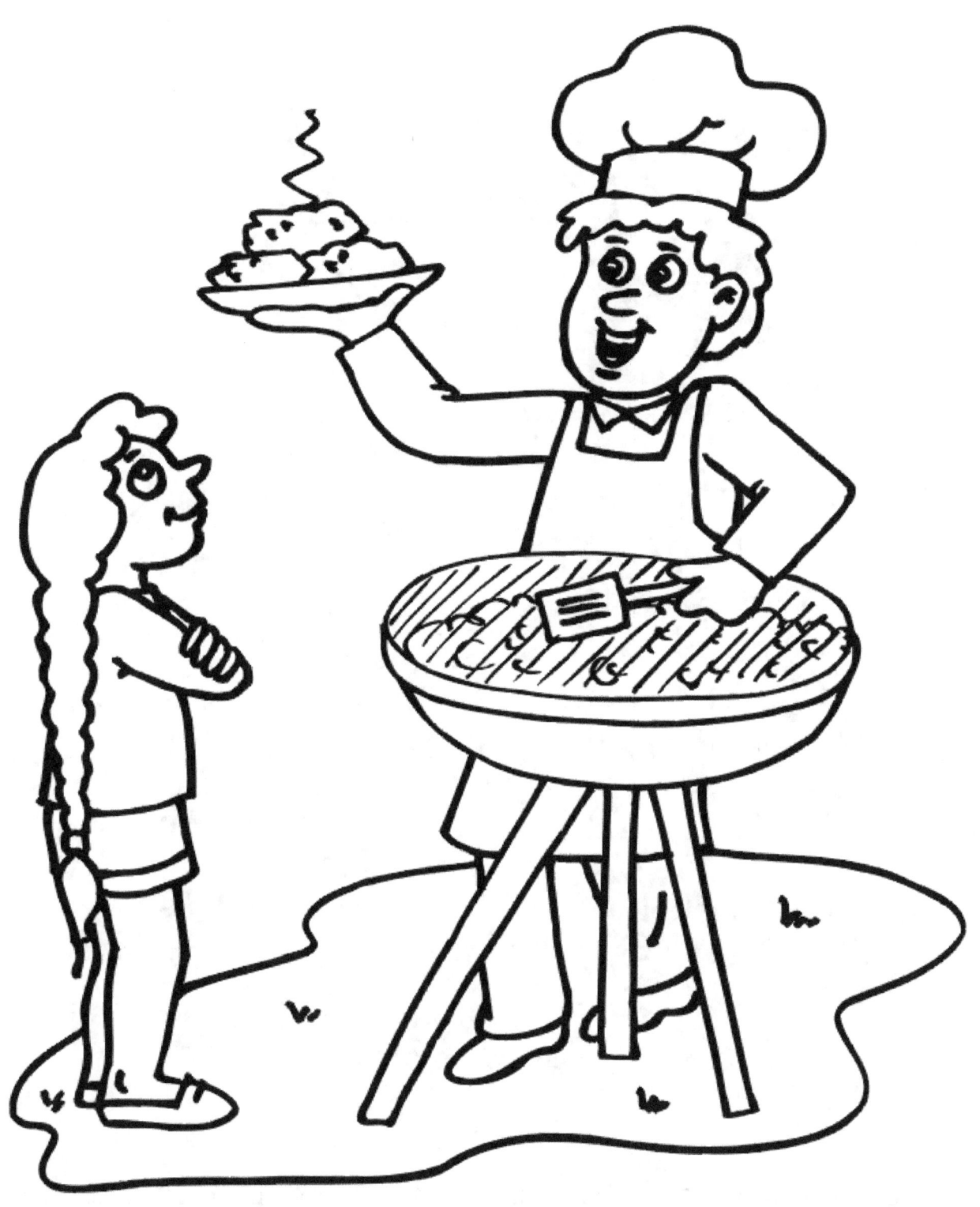

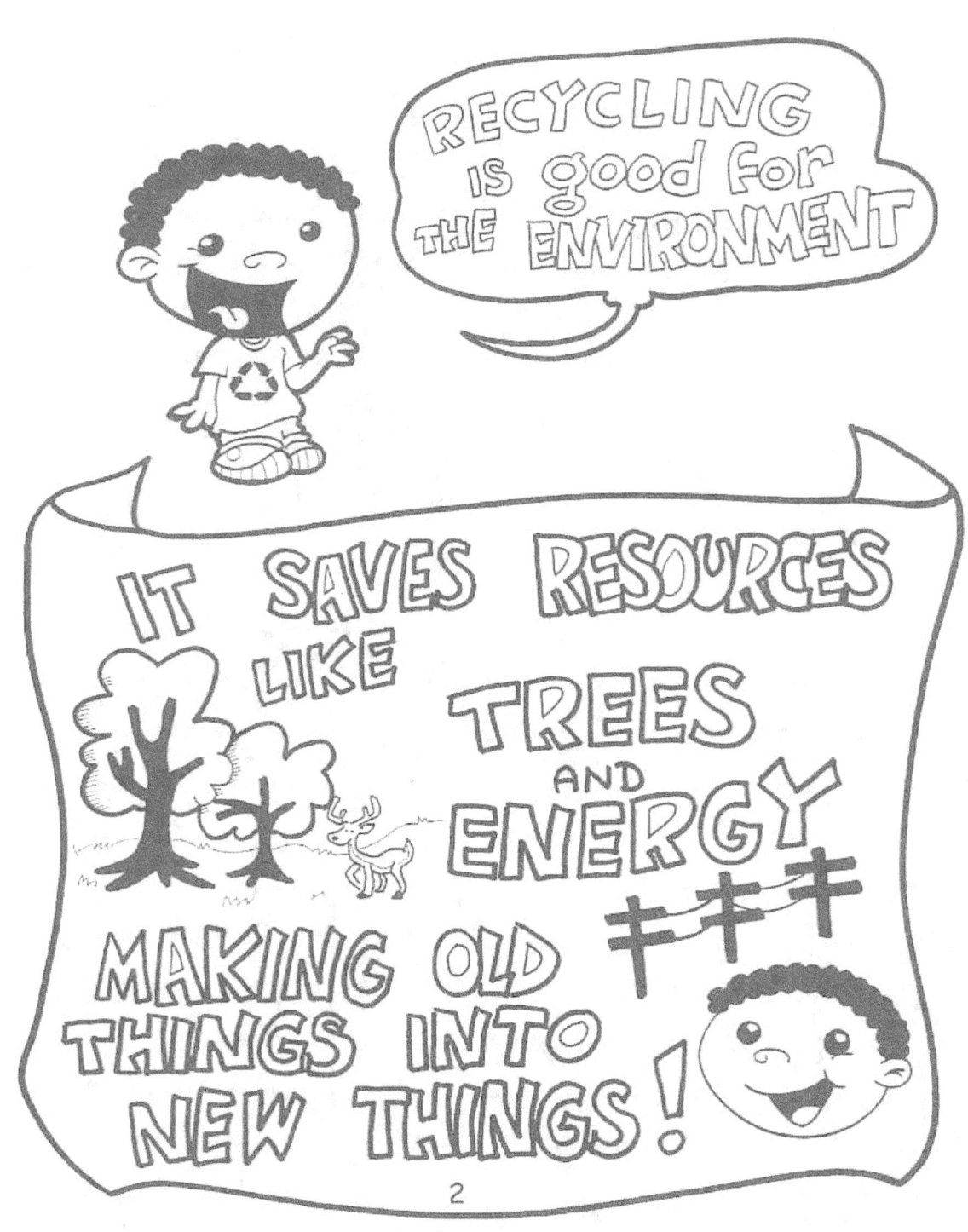

CAN YOU NAME **2** GOOD REASONS THAT WE SHOULD **RECYCLE** THINGS…?

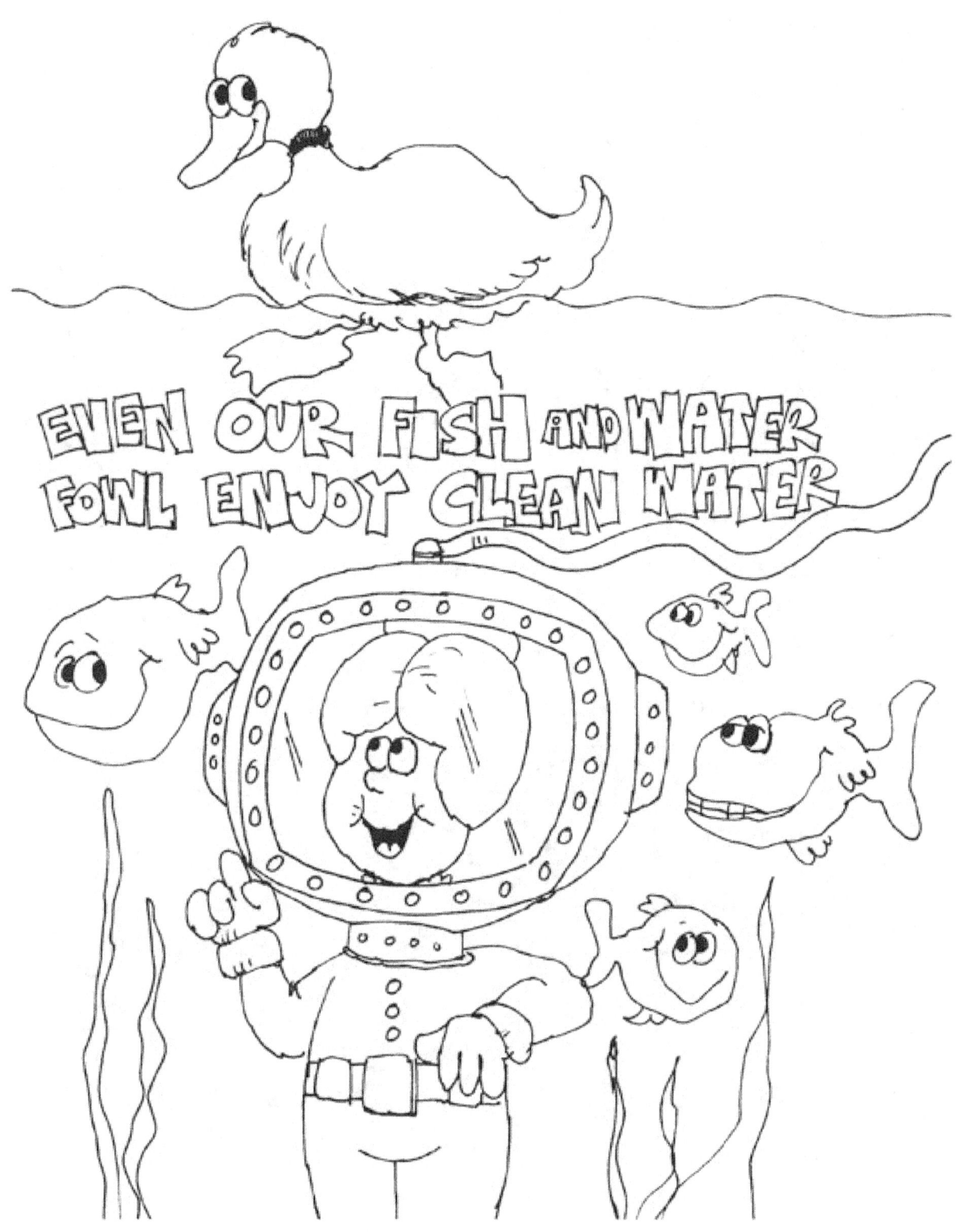

EVEN OUR FISH AND WATER FOWL ENJOY CLEAN WATER

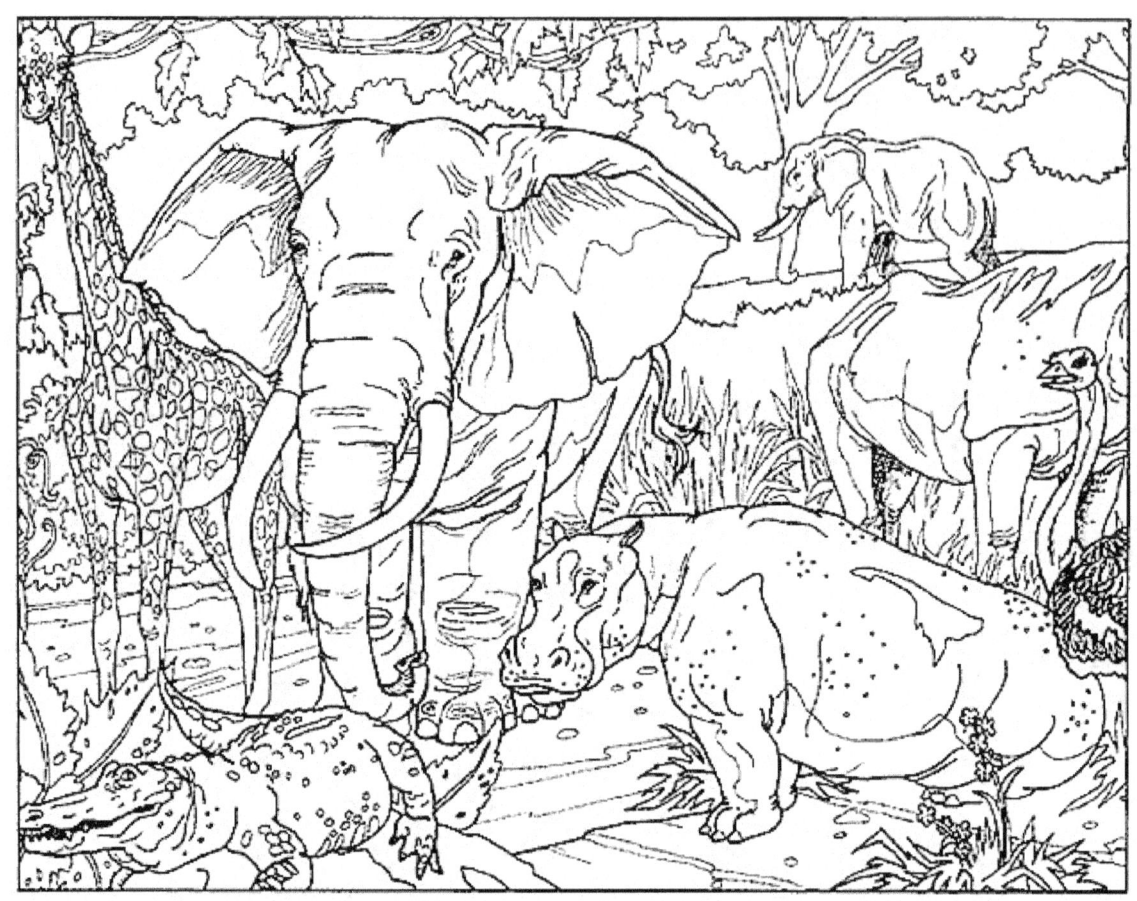

WHAT ANIMALS CAN YOU FIND IN THIS PICTURE?

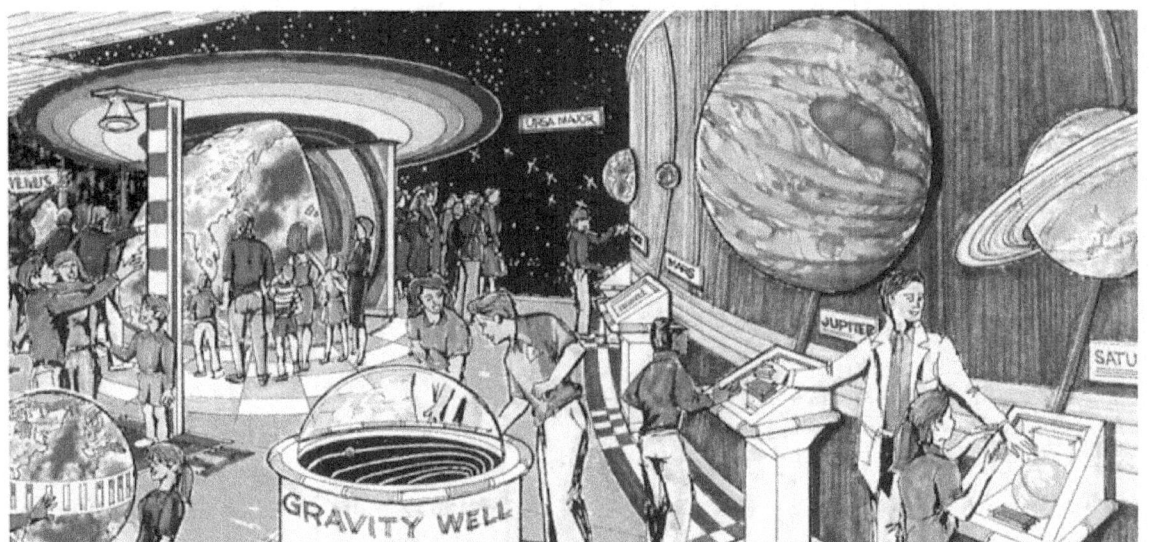

Learn more about our universe and thus -- about your own self.

NATURE WALK

Take this sheet with you while you go on a nature walk with family and friends.

Find a fallen leaf on the ground. Match it to one of these leaves to discover what kind of tree it belonged to. If your leaf is not one of the ones below, than draw a picture of it and look it up when you get home.

Oak

Pine

Maple

Look for bugs on the ground, on trees, or under rocks. Draw a picture of them here.

What animals have you seen on your walk? Draw a picture of them here:

There are many ways you can help the earth. List some ideas here:

_____

_____

_____

_____

_____

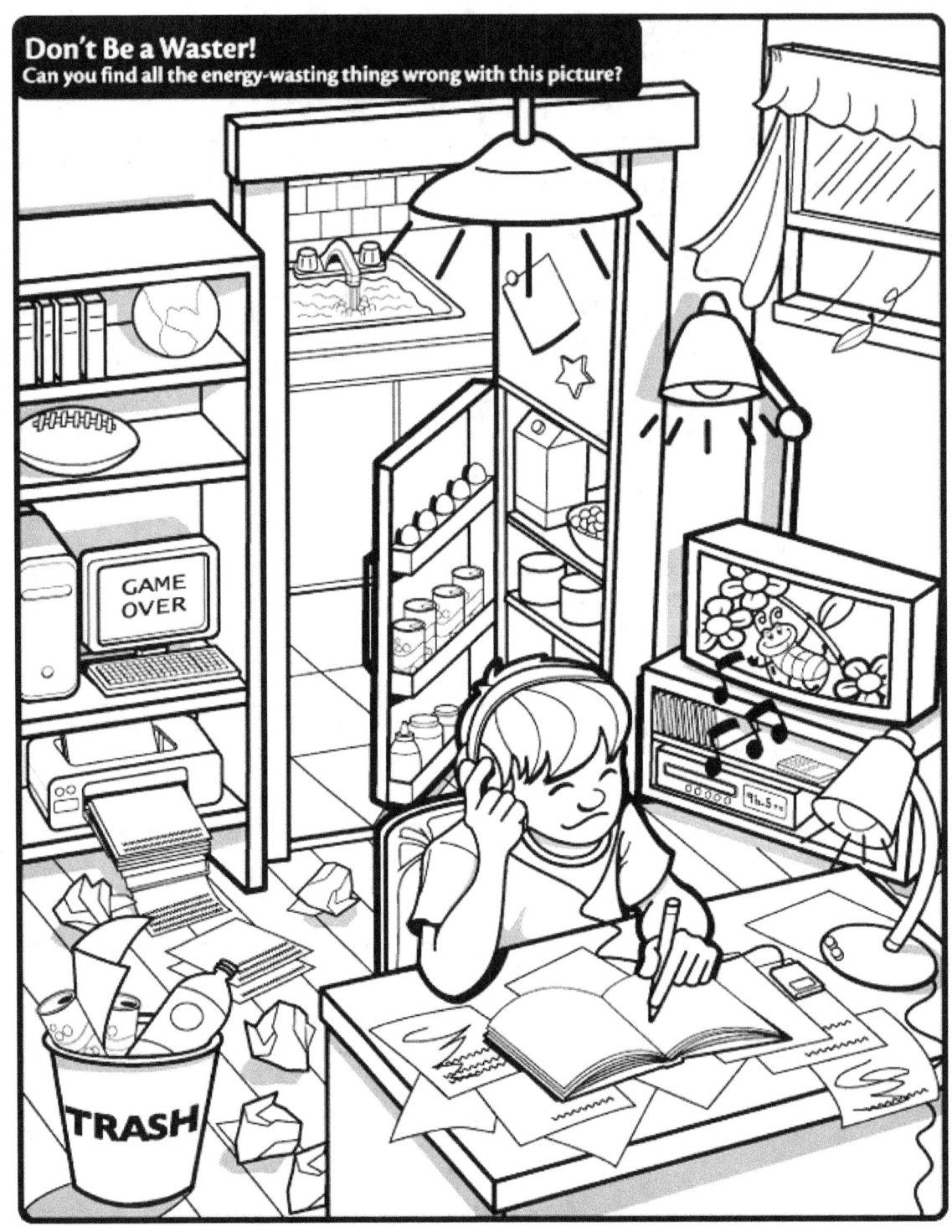

Color this picture and then make a list of ways this boy can save energy and <u>not</u> be so **wasteful.**

BOOKS FOR YOUTH

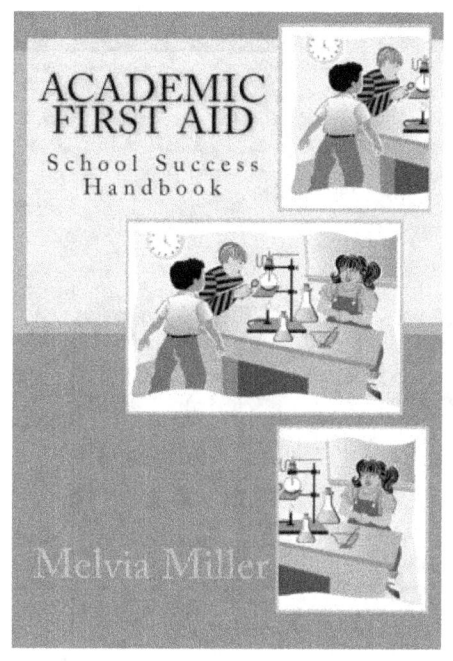

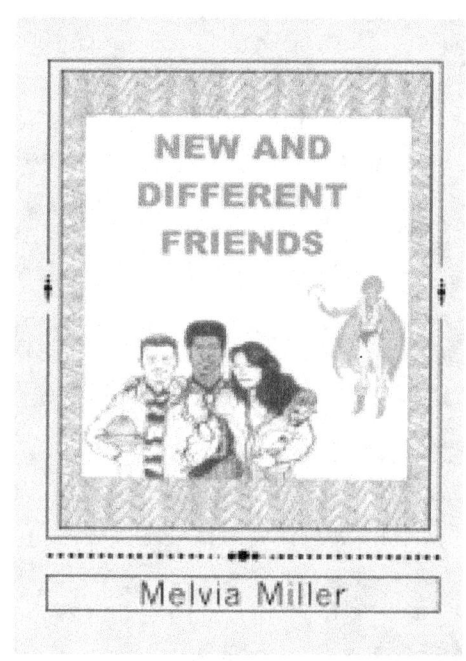

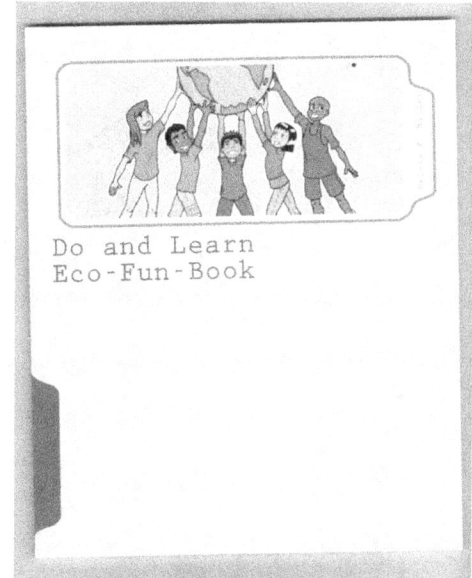

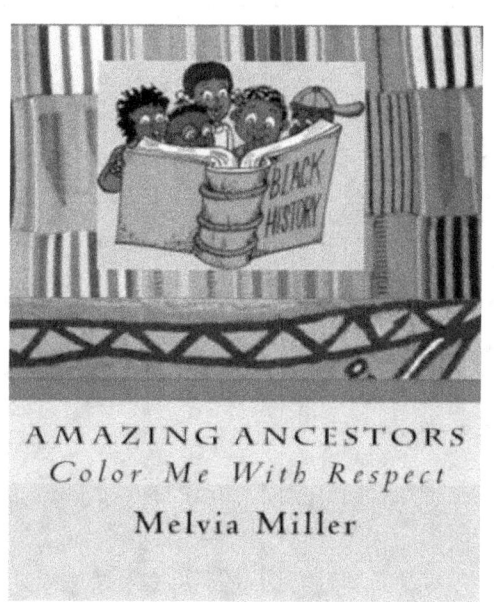

WWW.SUCCESS-SECRETS.WS

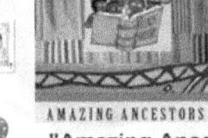 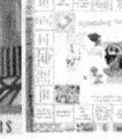
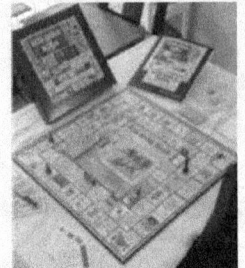 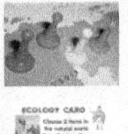 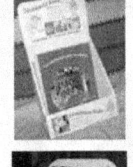 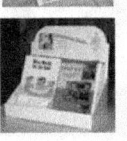 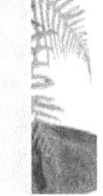
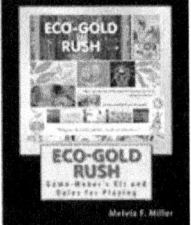
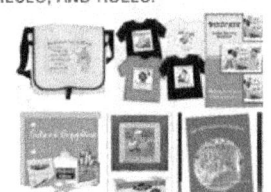
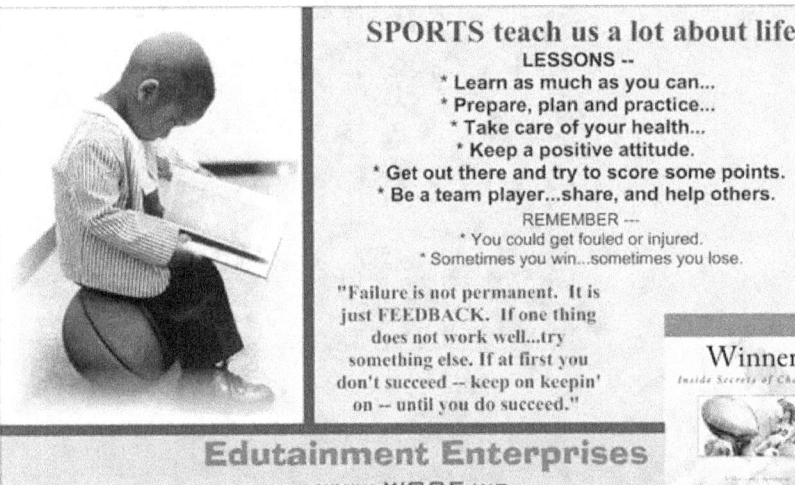
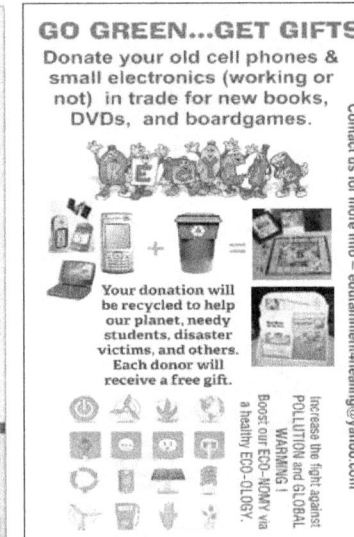

Edutainment Enterprises

GAMES, BOOKS,
DVDs, HEALTH
PRODUCTS,
OPPORTUNITIES...
AND MUCH MORE !

DISCOUNTS:
Any 3 books (B/W) @ $33.00
or any 3 full color books @ $55.00

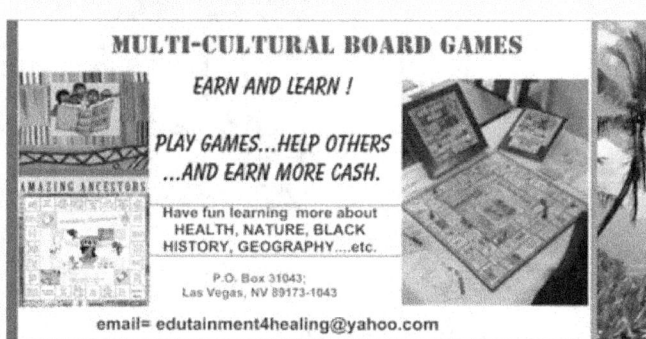

MULTI-CULTURAL BOARD GAMES

EARN AND LEARN !

*PLAY GAMES...HELP OTHERS
...AND EARN MORE CASH.*

Have fun learning more about
HEALTH, NATURE, BLACK
HISTORY, GEOGRAPHY....etc.

P.O. Box 31043;
Las Vegas, NV 89173-1043

email= edutainment4healing@yahoo.com

www.success-secrets.ws

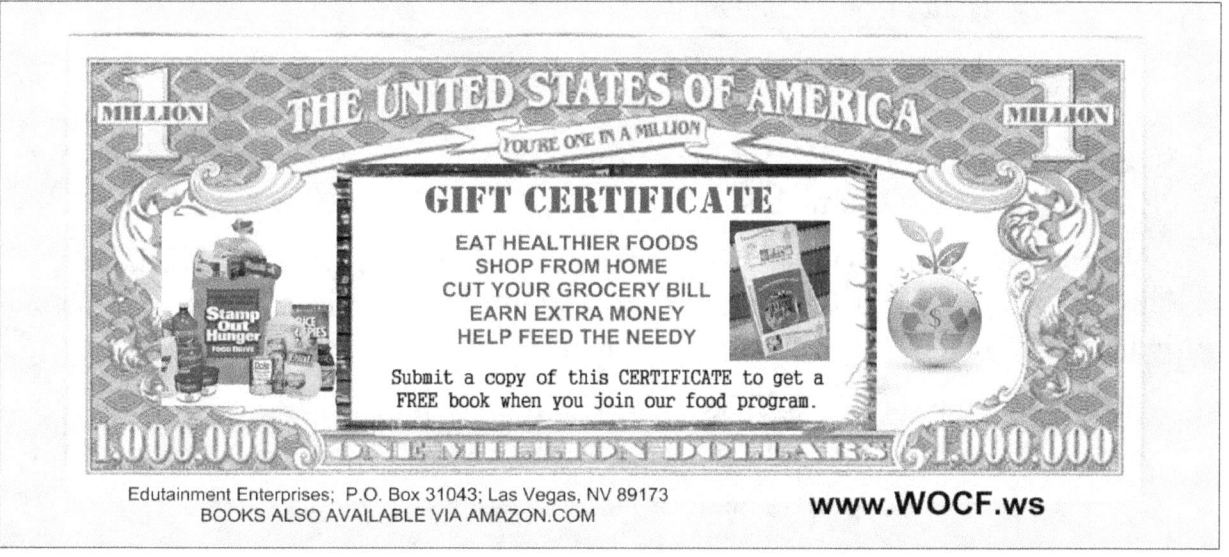

ABOUT THE AUTHOR

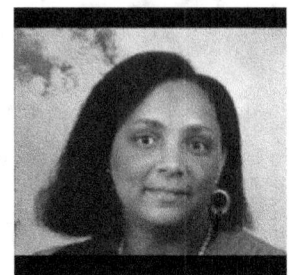
Melvia Miller

Melvia Miller is an educator/author who has created unique ways of teaching and training. She taught in public schools and colleges, and developed these unique materials based upon the concept of *"more effective and enjoyable training"* — **EDUTAINMENT.**

Having worked in major corporations as a manager, she also has experience in various aspects of seminars and business training ...and an excellent background in several areas. Other books by this author include:

- *The Virus Defense Handbook*
- *Edutainment Game Book*
- *Amazing Ancestors*

She also designed and produced unique board games and informative fun Edutainment DVD seminars.

With an excellent background in teaching, training, writing, publishing, and management, she offers stories and fables that delight the heart and enlighten our minds...help increase the peace!

Melvia is the mother of 2 sons: **Malik** and **Mikal.**

CONTACT by email - cultural-diversity@hotmail.com